SHAKEN BUT NOT STIRRED

All profits from this book will go to 'European Parkinson Therapy Centre' (www.parkinsontherapy.com), a non-profit advanced centre offering multilevel therapy for families and people with Parkinson's to help them 'take back their lives'.

Shaken but not Stirred

Amusing antidotes to a life with Parkinson's

Compiled by Alexander Reed and Dirma Van Toorn

Cartoons by Ron Leishman

Published by the European Parkinson's Therapy Centre
www.parkinsonitaly.com
Email: info@parkinsontherapy.com

Copyright © 2021 European Parkinson's Therapy Centre

The moral rights of the authors have been asserted

ISBN: 9798483844389

All rights reserved. No part of this publication may be reproduced, stored in any retrieval system, or transmitted, in any form or by any means, electronic, mechanical, photocopying, recording or otherwise, without the prior written permission of the publishers.

For all those who dedicate their lives to helping people with Parkinson's and their families.

Praise by Tom Isaacs

Tom Isaacs is the President and Co-founder of *The Cure Parkinson's Trust*.

When you have Parkinson's it is important that you live your life as a 'glass half-full' sort of person – but that's because you tend to spill the rest!

Shaken but not Stirred is an essential tool for all people who live or work with Parkinson's. Not only does it demonstrate that humour can be found even in the murky depths of a degenerative neurological condition, but the book also illustrates that living 'well' is about attitude not circumstance.

Expect to experience a full spectrum of emotions as you read these short stories. But, at the end, I guarantee you will come away with a warm and cosy feeling that life isn't that bad and, hey, you might even enjoy yourself a little bit!

Tom

Praise by Dr Michele Hu

Dr Michele Hu is an Associate Professor in the Department of Clinical Neurology at *the Nuffield Department of Clinical Neurosciences, University of Oxford* and Consultant Neurologist at *Oxford University Hospitals*. She is chairperson of the Research Engagement sub-committee of the *UK Parkinson's Excellence Network* and Co-Principal Investigator of the *Oxford Parkinson's Disease Centre*.

The quality of empathy, defined in the *Oxford Advanced Learner's Dictionary* as 'the ability to understand and share the feelings of another', is key to the doctor-patient relationship. However, unless you have gone through the experience of being diagnosed and coming to terms with Parkinson's yourself, your personal understanding will be limited. Health professionals and all those involved with the care of people with Parkinson's will therefore benefit tremendously from this book, which is at times hilarious, quirky and moving. A series of light-hearted, real life short stories written by individuals who have gone through the journey of dealing with Parkinson's make this book unique, insightful and practical.

This book will be highly valuable for people who are newly diagnosed with Parkinson's, people struggling with the condition, family members and anybody who wants to truly understand and get alongside the person with Parkinson's. I am delighted to be able to recommend this highly to you.

Dr Michele Hu

Foreword by Richard Curtis

Richard is a comedy writer and director whose credits include Love Actually, Notting Hill, Four Weddings and a Funeral, About Time, Blackadder and Mr Bean.

One of the contributors to this book happens to be an old friend, and although Paul Mayhew-Archer is a 'person with Parkinson's', in all other respects he is the same person he ever was, with the same love of classical music, the same penchant for enormous bars of whole nut chocolate, the same eccentric collection of jumpers and above all the same sense of fun. We worked together on *The Vicar of Dibley* and *Esio Trot* and those are the two happiest jobs I ever did in my life.

Parkinson's is of course a 'serious illness', and the trouble with serious illnesses is that when people get a serious illness we all tend to become very serious about it. Too frequently we give them seriously sympathetic looks and we say, 'How are you?' in our most serious voice. And we tell our friends, 'Old so-and-so's got Parkinson's or cancer or a brain tumour' and they say,

'Oh no, that's serious. Do you remember the laughs we used to have?' and we say, 'Oh yes, old so-and-so was a great laugh.' And we chuckle at the memory until one of us says, 'Still, all good things must come to an end,' and we look all serious again.

So this book is a lovely little reminder that a serious illness does not have to be taken entirely seriously. Yes, there will be moments when 'laughing in the aisles' is inappropriate - when an injection is being administered, for example, or during the funeral - but much of the time illness can be funny and we will all feel better for laughing at it. I've nursed both my Mum and Dad and we always tried to keep enjoying ourselves. When my Dad had really forgotten everything, my Mum and I saw the funny side of it, and laughter, which had always been central in our family life, kept its place at the table.

So here's to chuckling at an incurable neurological disease. And here's hoping that, as Paul's Parkinson's progresses, he forgets where he left all his jumpers (he is SO wrong – purple doesn't go with everything) and has to buy some new ones. I'm serious.

Richard Curtis

CONTENTS

Chapter One - Dirma | p. 15

Chapter Two - Sally | p. 71

Chaptesr Three - Richard | p. 83

Chapter Four - John | p. 93

Chapter Five - Paul | p. 107

Chapter Six - Alex | p. 121

Chapter Seven - Humphrey | p. 153

Chapter Eight - Andrew and Esther | p. 163

Conclusion | p. 177

References | p. 187

Chapter One
Dirma

Dirma van Toorn

Dirma was born in 1958 in Quelderland, Holland. She now lives in Media City Hilversum with her husband and her daughter.
In 1999 Dirma's mother was diagnosed with Alzheimer's, so Dirma and her family decided to take her into their home, and Dirma had to say goodbye to her job and career. Her mother died suddenly in 2003 from a fatal brain haemorrhage, and directly after her death Dirma started to develop the then-unknown symptoms of Parkinson's, although the official diagnosis didn't come until two years later.
She decided to commit her daily obstacles with Parkinson's to paper. Her first book 'Pee en ik' was successfully published in Holland. She also writes poems and scripts for theatre and film. Two children's books are also on their way.

Dirma's stories relate to P (Parkinson's) as a thinking and often mischievous being whose life with the author leads to greater insight into who P really is.

The translation of these stories from Dutch to English was done with the help of Pete Hotchkin.

P&I
Becoming suspects

I had finally managed to get my husband to accompany me into town. Not that I needed a chaperone, but it was almost Christmas, and the thought of terrible queues at the tills already had me hyperventilating.

After some self-sacrifice and mumbling something to do with women and Christmas, my husband agreed, and so our adventure began.

A dark cloud appeared, and I hoped we would be able to get to the shops before the heavens opened. I had forgotten to put my good shoes on and also had my Yeti extra thick and warm (but horrendously ugly) jacket, but it was too late to get changed so we set off with some speed.

We agreed that I would look for the presents whilst my husband grabbed a place in the long checkout queue. I believe that all men detest shopping – it's in their DNA – but he dutifully took his place, and I set off to seriously lighten his wallet by my return.

Great start but, as if he was in a conspiracy with my husband to limit my enthusiasm to spend, P made his move. My arms became like wooden sticks and I

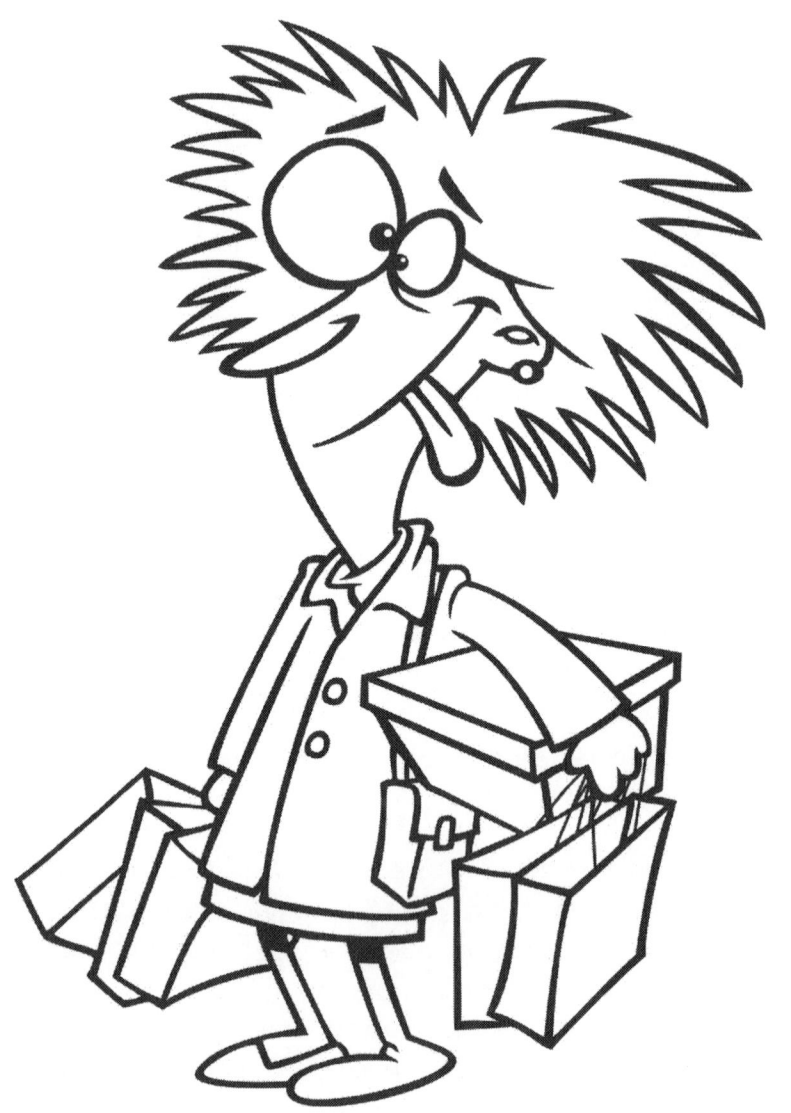

hid my hands away as P started his shaking routine. P does so like to appear at inconvenient moments. I could almost see him smiling.

On top of that, I looked a mess, partly due to the odd shoes and jacket, and partly because I had forgotten to put any makeup on. At least that morning, with the help of a cloud of chemicals, I had been able to squash my hair down, which had been leading its own life recently. With my trash-style look and P doing his 'I'm a shaking, wobbling mad' routine, I must have been quite a sight. Clearly the personnel and security guard in the shop noticed, and, sure enough, a suspicious assistant came over and enquired, 'Are you looking for something?'

With a straight face and swaying from left to right, I said, 'Not really, I'm just looking around'. So, as if to demonstrate my sincerity, I did start looking around me. Indeed, I turned so suddenly that I almost fell into the arms of a security guard.

After trying to smile at the man, I stiffened under his serious gaze. In all fairness, I had been walking like a zombie along the rows and rows of decoratively displayed goods. I was without a handbag and, due to P's influence, I had my hands stuffed in my pockets! Naturally the suspicious sales lady thought that I wanted to steal something, and the security guard appeared to have reached the same conclusion. When I had come in, he had been standing mainly near the front door, but now he was following me around like a dog, almost panting, and with that blissful look such people get when they are ready to arrest someone. He had never heard of P.

Sometime later, and with my arms full of whatnots and knickknacks, I trudged towards the till and my husband, who appeared on the verge of making a run for it. I handed over the goods and tried to ignore his muttering of, 'Couldn't you find any more stuff?' He stood in the queue whilst P and I stood to one side near the exit.

No doubt this also looked suspicious, as they came to check on me one more time to make sure we were not running off with the loot. The image of me making a run for it with P wobbling along beside me was too much to take in and I burst out laughing. The security guard had no idea how to take this and watched menacingly as P and I made a shuffling retreat from his gaze into the street where P surprisingly decided to take a back seat as I walked smoothly away from the shop.

P&I
A traitor in our midst

That day I made a life-changing decision: it was time to tackle my daughter's room! The piles of clothes and books that littered the floor left no room to actually see the floor. I had not planned to become her slave, but I could no longer deny the mess, or the gentle wafting of a smell that I could only describe as being… well, smelly. So whether or not P agreed with me, that day I was going to be like Hercules and do it.

I went upstairs in a really good mood. I threw open the door and worked out my plan of attack. Yes, I was going to start by sorting out the school books from the reading books, and separating the dirty clothes from the clean ones to put away. I could then make the bed and do the dusting and vacuuming tomorrow.

Good plan… but I forgot one tiny detail.

P decided to help out too, but it soon became clear whose side he was on. P was sitting so heavily on my back that I couldn't stand up with books in my arms. If I leaned forward he gave me a push so that I would fall sideways, and if I tried to reach up to move things on top of the wardrobe he'd make my arms ache, so I just sat down and shouted at the world. I got really angry with P.

A new plan was required. I had a traitor in my ranks. P anticipated my every move, or more precisely he was stopping my every move. Like a general in a war zone I had to use cunning to trick him into a false sense of security. So I went for the strategy of sitting down and letting P think he was winning, then I would move stealthily and push a book here and a sock there before stopping again so that he wouldn't realise what I was doing.

It took me two days, but in the end I made it, maybe not like Hercules – more like his pet snail with asthma.

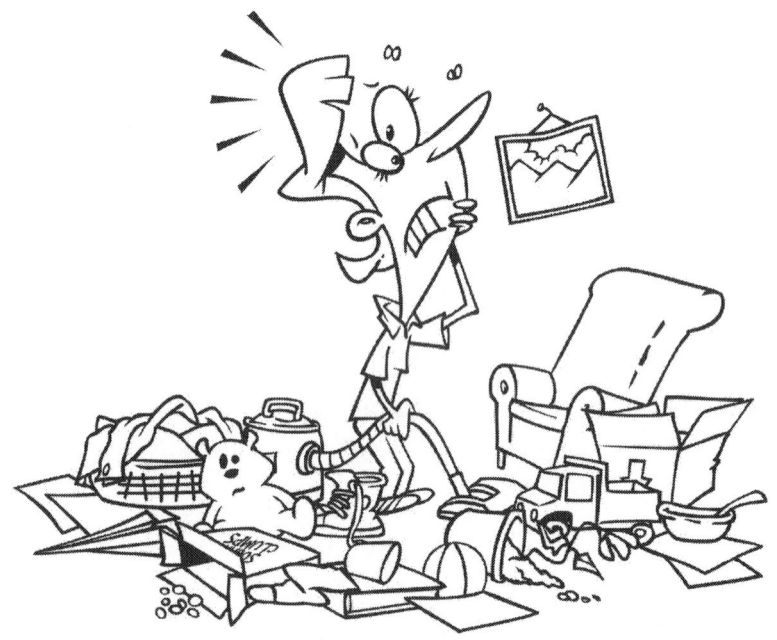

A great victory, I thought as I walked up the stairs some days later, and like all great victories it should be savoured. So I slowly opened the door to my daughter's room, and realised that the real traitor was not P. Once again the floor had done a disappearing act, probably never to be seen again as I was greeted by the familiar smell of defeat.

P can be tricked, controlled and even told what to do on some occasions; daughters are a much greater challenge. I closed the door and decided to go to bed, which P finally agreed as being the best compromise.

P&I
A gardener's tale

It was early afternoon and I had decided to do something with the front garden. It was one of those rare days in May with good weather. There was a lovely warm breeze blowing, and I quietly opened the door, almost as if not to wake P.
'Good morning Mrs. T,' I span around in surprise, and there was my elderly neighbour with spade in hand, wearing some kind of coat which reminded me vaguely of my grandmother.

'How are you this morning?' he shouted. Ah, the inescapable daily routine of the greeting and the small talk. I would have loved to reply that P kept me up all night and that he had come up with a new trick, which he found terribly funny, of occasionally moving my hand or leg such that when walking down the street I received several waves and numerous hellos, as people mistook my elaborate hand movements for a form of greeting.

I replied, 'Absolutely fine thank you,' and P gave him a wave.

I moved on, still waving, to my garden.

DIRMA

Right, where shall I start?

Ivy was growing rampantly throughout the whole garden. Some of the bushes had grown into each other so you could not see where one started and the other finished. Many leaves had fallen during the dry period and they were still lying on the grass. The borders were also a mess. The daisies were almost knee high. The beech trees had not finished flowering and they were dropping pollen everywhere – on the post box, on the windowsills, etc. The edging stones, which were supposed to separate the grass from the gravel,

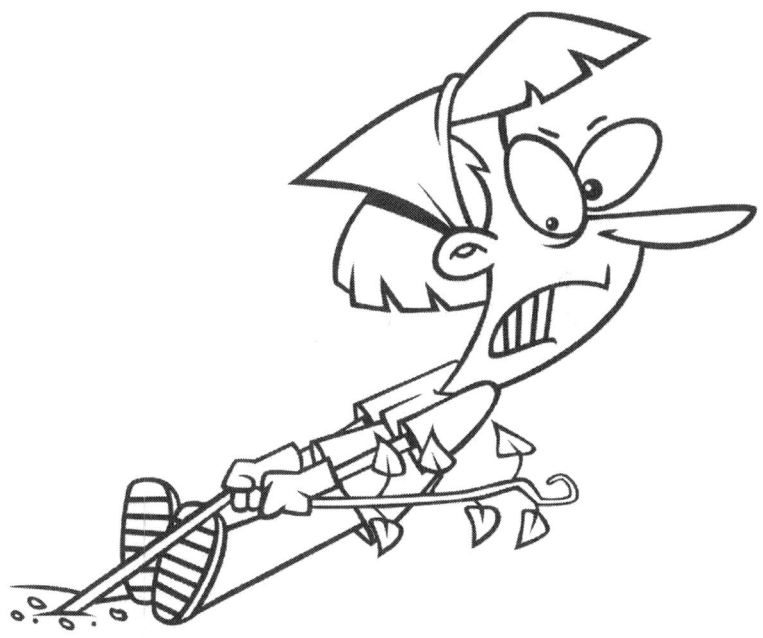

were no longer visible. The grass had cheekily grown over them and at least 10 centimetres over the gravel. You may have guessed by now that I have never been a great gardener.

The hidden stones intrigued me, and I decided to begin with them.

During my inspection, I had completely forgotten about P. I managed to get down nicely onto my knees without falling over. It was hard work, but I progressed quite quickly and I was almost finished after an hour. I then decided to move some logs, and my 87 year old neighbour came to help me with the sawing. Shouldn't it be the other way round?

But where the heck had P gone?

It was now three thirty. The sun had given way to clouds, and it looked likely to start raining soon. I had to hurry up.

It was really lovely being in the garden. I felt like my old self again. It was rather strange though; I missed P. He is such a big part of me that it feels weird not having him around sometimes. No, that was crazy. I must have been going crazy.

I decided to take a break at half past five, and I was just thinking that I could have had a go on mowing the lawn next when a young lad came by trying to sell me some pens. I tried to get back into the house to get some change for him, when I suddenly realised that I had accidentally managed to lock myself out! The boy shrugged his shoulders at my sudden rush of panic and I gave an involuntary wave of the hand. Ooops… P was back. He then moved my other hand, and like a symphony conductor I started flapping my hands in all directions. The boy by now was mesmerized and not sure whether to wave back or make a run for it. Fortunately my husband arrived, and seeing the boy's predicament he calmly explained, 'It's all right, it's her Parkinson's'. The boy made a run for it anyway!

P&I
Deep pockets

For the first time in ages the weather was decent, and P was silent, which meant my hand tremor was absent too.

The sun emerged carefully from behind the clouds, and I felt that spring had arrived at last. Winter had delayed it by lasting twice as long as usual. Finally I could go and walk the dog without the need of my beloved, baggy coat!

When the sun shines we always have something of a battle, P and I. I exclaim, 'What a beautiful day, today!' but P trudges along ahead of me, sulking.

Now, should I go on the road or on the path through the woods? P and I chose the woods. Five minutes later, P whispered into my ear that I had forgotten my coat. 'Ha ha,' I thought, 'No problem – I don't need it today,' but then it dawned on me… winter coat equalled deep pockets… ahhh… the pockets! A Parkinson's escape route when tremor strikes - and I had left them behind.

Despite my predicament the dog still needed his walk, so I decided to carry on. But I suddenly had the nudging feeling that this was not going to be my day after all and that P had set me up. I was right, of course.

150 metres ahead I saw someone walking towards me. I thought about running away, but P did not let me. With no chance of escape, I suddenly felt P starting to make my hand tremble, so I jumped into a bush to hide. Clever idea Dirma… I had outwitted P, as whoever it was would never find me here…

'Good morning Mrs T. How are you today?'

It was my neighbour, asking that stupid question again. Busted!

'Fine,' I replied. 'Just dropped something.'

At that moment, another voice shouted out, 'Frank, why are you talking to that bush?'

Great, so now there were two of them.

'That's no bush, it's my neighbour who just dropped something!'

I decided to come out from my useless hiding place and, as suspected, P increased even further my hand shaking. I had no pockets, I had no coat, I had no escape route. So I did the next best thing and stuck my hand down my trousers.

With mud streaking my face, leaves clinging to my shirt and one hand down my trousers, I was truly the victim of P's manipulation, and he once again succeeded in making me look like a complete idiot. Perfect, just perfect!

P & I
Brushes, lipsticks and eyeliners

Brushing my teeth was something I never had to think about even for one second. I used to stand in front of the mirror, and whilst I removed my breakfast from between my teeth, I would to go through my plans for the day. I would whizz the brush at high speed over my teeth and gums, and not give it a second thought, humming away to whatever tune had got stuck in my head that morning.

Easy, right? Wrong.

P gradually took an interest in my morning brushing ritual. He obviously didn't like my humming as he forced me to focus all of my attention on the toothbrush so that doing anything else was not an option anymore. Yet, whilst he didn't interfere with the up and down movement, he didn't like the side to side one, and it was this that became the battle ground between us.

Why wasn't the toothbrush behaving like I wanted it to? The answer was of course P. When the battle was finally over it felt good to have teeth glimmering back at me and a nose half covered in toothpaste.

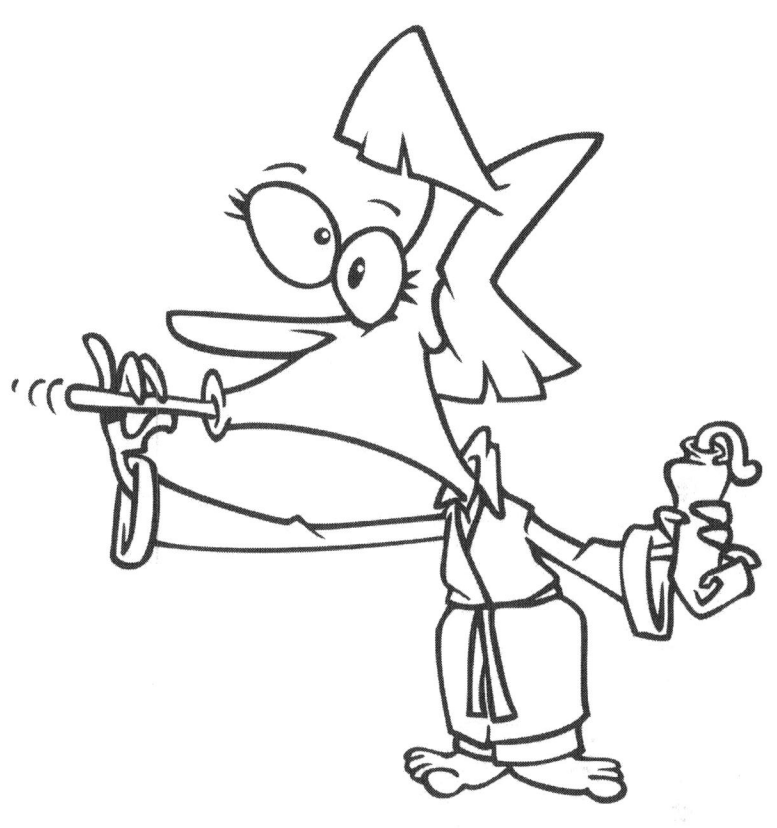

P has taught me a lot over the years, the biggest thing being that you should never give up, just find an alternative solution. So I found a way to outwit P by buying an electric toothbrush and learning the joys of whirling heads and buzzing handles.

But P's curiosity and desire to 'get involved' did not stop with my teeth. Face painting soon became his new hobby. On other people without P, that would be called putting your make up on. One evening we went to a party and P had done such a good job that I ended up with eyeliner on my forehead, and the lipstick... Well, I won't tell you were that ended up.

Brushing my hair was, even before P, like taming a wild jungle. P turned it into a hopeless farce, and the best I could do was achieve a sort of bundle that floated on top of my head.

This may have given the impression that I looked slightly odd, and my new gypsy look was certainly noticed by my friends, one of whom actually tried to fix things. That really agitated P and he refused to go out that evening, employing his favourite trick of increasing the tremor in my hand to the extent that eating with that hand was like an egg and spoon race where the egg always falls off.

P and I have now come to an arrangement. If during the year he lets me use very little make-up, once every twelve months P may do anything he wants with my face: when it is Carnival. He is allowed do all my make-up on that day. I don't care about what colours he chooses, how much make-up he uses or where my lipstick ends up. This way we both have fun.

P & I
A Christmas tale

Soon after the leaves had fallen and the warm sunny days had turned into long chilly nights, the Christmas tree was decorated, no thanks to P but to a long-suffering husband who got reluctantly persuaded into hanging baubles and lights. We put the Christmas tree in its standard position in the bay window, and with the sound of Bach's *Christmas Oratorio* in the background, we initiated the festive season.

And so began the yearly ritual of sending cards to people you hardly ever meet, and some who you will meet very soon but need a card for anyhow.

Correspondence should always look perfect. That was not up for discussion. However, beautiful handwriting was, unfortunately, a talent that I never possessed. P turns poor handwriting into a scribble so that the words I put together on paper with such care are in fact totally illegible.

I pushed on, with P still giving my elbow a nudge and making my handwriting so small that it would be quicker to draw a straight line. It ended up becoming a complete warzone. Big letters turned into little letters, little letters became squiggly letters, and then suddenly a big scratch.

The cards truly were a problem. I was always a fierce opponent of 'Senders'. These are the people who send way too many cards purely to sign their name on them – nothing else, nothing about themselves, nothing about you. Just a very impersonal signature, almost as if they were documents from the bank.

When it came to putting the cards in the envelopes, I inserted one corner first and started to insert the second one whilst P pulled out the first. P scarcely ever gives up but I do: I ended up just stuffing the cards in as quickly as possible.

At this point I silently offered up my apologies to the many receivers who get crumpled cards from me and who probably don't even know they are from me in first place since there is never anything legible inside!

More recently I've adopted a more direct approach. I pick up the phone and wish 'Merry Christmas', even to those who have to ask me twice who I am.

P&I
Contact!

That day I got my new contact lenses! Finally no more glasses, and especially no more losing the stupid things.

I opened the box with great anticipation and there they were, glittering in the light. P and I were in the sitting room and P appeared calm and laid back, not even curious about the novelty. I placed myself in front of the sitting room mirror and, following the instructions, I used one finger of my right hand to gently place the left contact into my eye whilst holding up my eyelid with my left hand.

The inevitable then happened…. I had forgotten P was right handed, and with a little tremor of the hand the lens was lost! P wasn't curious, he was just plain mischievous. The lens had fallen into the shagpile carpet and was nowhere to be seen.

I dropped to my knees with P on my back and with shaky hands and my body trembling I searched carefully through the diabolical carpet. I found nothing! Oh P, what have you done! Where could that missing thing be? Worst still, I had left my glasses somewhere sensible but not logical, and everything looked blurred.

Plenty of curses came to mind. P jeered at them.

Now what? First I carefully removed the chairs, then the heavy old oak table. Then I had the ingenious idea of rolling up the carpet (which was almost too heavy to lift) and watching carefully with my very blurry vision to see if anything fell out, but to no avail.

At that moment, the doorbell rang, giving me quite a fright. Even P was silenced by it, and I walked over to the door, knocking off a picture on my way as I couldn't see without my glasses. Wrong door; I ended up greeting the vacuum cleaner in our downstairs closet. Next door to the right; yes, that was definitely the one. I opened it but all I could see was a fuzzy image, but no greeting was forthcoming and I feared I had made the terrible mistake of opening the door without asking who it was. A voice came out of the blur, 'Good morning Mrs. T, how are you this morning, could I bother you for some sugar?' It was my neighbour. And I gave the polite response, 'Sure, come in.' Then I remembered that behind me the carpet was pulled up, chairs were knocked over and a picture was lying on the floor. My once beautiful sitting room was a bombsite. 'Just doing a little spring cleaning'.

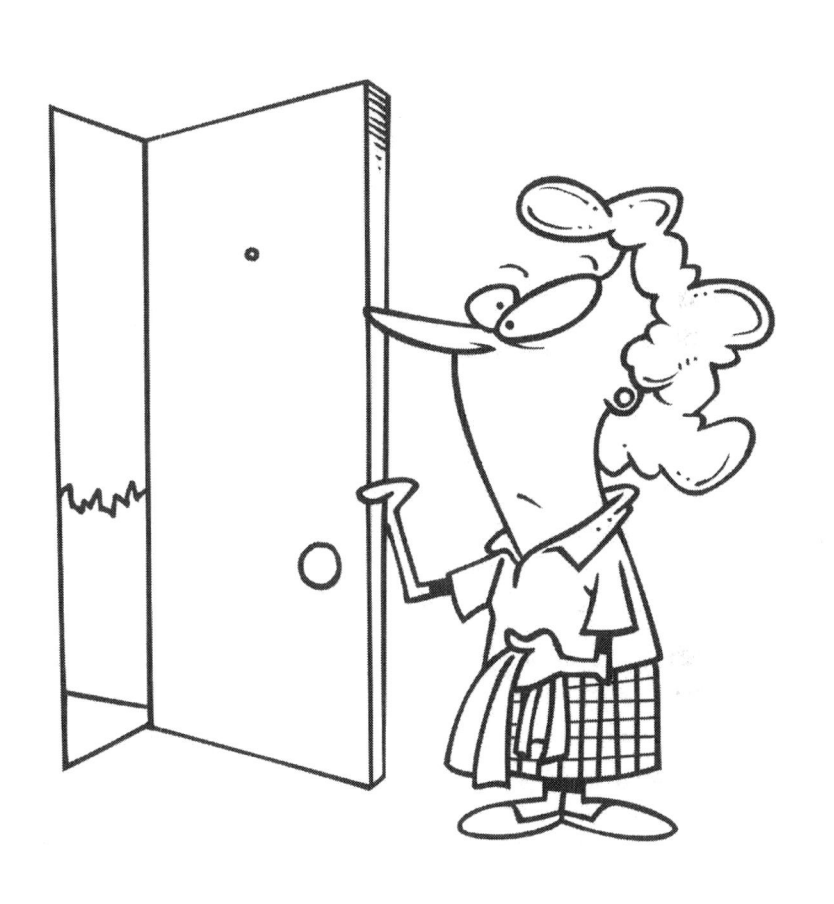

P&I
George and I

One sunny day, I was driving on the motorway en route to my friend's house in the south of the country. I had left early in the morning because it was a good one-and-a-half-hour journey. My hope not to get stuck in a traffic jam was misplaced, because Holland without traffic jams is unthinkable.

I had already given up a while back the idea of speeding along in the fast lane. It was too fast for me now. That day I had decided to stay behind a truck – nice and safe. Another truck had the same idea and placed itself behind me. And yet another was trying to overtake all three of us, but in reality it ended up beside me with a large bearded man peering down at me. I froze and looked straight ahead, searching for the nearest junction.

The truck driver behind me didn't try very hard to keep his distance and I could guess what he was thinking. I tried to pull out but bearded man left no space. When he finally allowed some extra space for me to pass, I put my foot on the gas and, with a sigh of relief, I shot out and down the line of trucks. P just sat on the seat and pulled faces at truck drivers and passers-by, causing lots of them to stare in with angry surprise. Where had the time gone since my friend and I tore down to the South of France in an old VW Beetle and where, in the middle of the night, we got to drive a Corniche between Nice and Monaco, just for the thrill of the bends?

Finally I got to my exit and I swung across the lanes, just like the old days back in France. P was silent – terrified I think; finally I had the power to silence him.

Somebody else was in a terrible rush. It was a good-looking guy and I looked closer, intrigued. If you half closed your eyes he could have been George Clooney in a Mercedes. Hoooonk, hooonk... Oops, I didn't let him pass, so I opened my eyes wide again. George certainly didn't look pleased.

P shot him a wave – well why not? He was good looking, although certainly not George Clooney. He shot me a hand signal, which was not a greeting and not something George would ever do!

When I finally arrived at my destination, my friend was already waiting outside.

'You are just in time, my brother is just about to arrive, he so wanted to meet you, but he called me to say he was a little late because of some idiot who tried to cut him up on the motorway, and even had the cheek to wave.'

Indeed, slowly up the drive came a Mercedes with a not very smiling George!

P&I
Dance the night away

When I was young I used to love dancing and partying till the small hours. I was thinking about my misspent youth and reflecting on the fact that today I would not get away with doing the boogie-woogie – it would look more like the 'shaky flakey'. Where had those great times suddenly disappeared to?

I still went dancing, but I found that my body did not respond exactly in time with the beat. That short millisecond delay between hearing the beat and my muscles responding to it was the difference between great dancing and an embarrassing shuffle. P didn't like dancing and was the main cause of this reversal of artistic prowess. All I had inherited from my musical father had fled long ago on its heels.

Even so, I decided to persevere and regain some of the boogie if not the woogie.

One weekend I downloaded some old music, thinking that, with the combination of memories and the music, I could make P love dancing.

I put on a waltz by Lehar. I stood up, put P in a corner and felt light as a feather as I glided over the

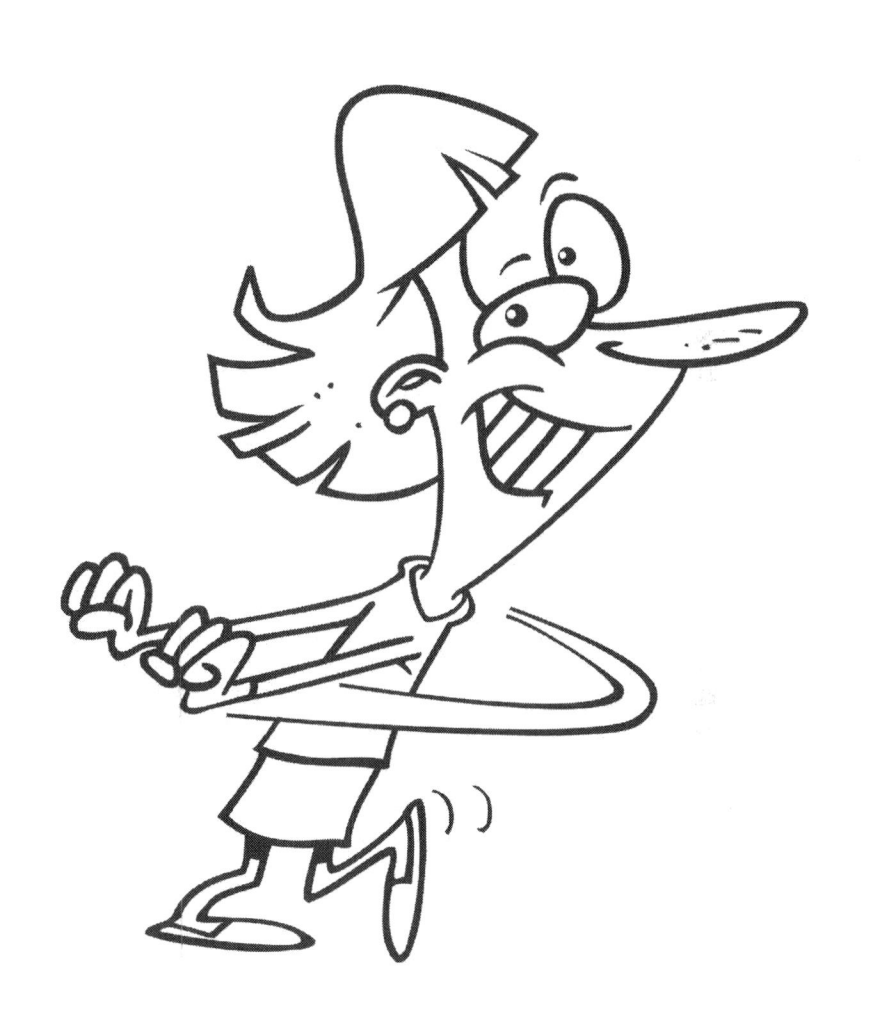

wooden floor. I danced through the room with a perfect feeling for timing and rhythm. What a surprise, I could still do the waltz!

Armed with this new wave of enthusiasm, I convinced my husband to sign up for classic dancing twice a week.

Our first night was a disaster. No, P could not be blamed with this one. My husband's two left feet left me bruised and battered.

So now P and I go dancing. P sits in the corner and sulks, whilst I glide over the dance floor with any man who will have me.

P&I
Orange bitter

The next day was Queen's Day in Holland and we were planning a party. P was getting very excited. Parties meant lots of opportunities for causing mayhem. Therefore, that day we really had to get all the shopping done. Fully aware that P did not like shopping, I wrote down the shopping list to avoid coming home with only half of what we needed.

Off we set to the supermarket, all three of us. Me, my husband and P.

Good planning always helps when P is around. But leaving the list behind was not part of the plan.

Ok, no panic. I told myself to keep calm and to keep breathing normally. I could remember all the items on that list, so I could make it.

Luckily, it all went like clockwork, and soon I had lots of delightful delicacies in my shopping trolley. It would be a great party, and all our guests deserved to be spoilt.

The lady behind the till asked me whether I needed any help packing up all the shopping. Well, I certainly couldn't turn down this offer, as it took P out of the equation and sped up our departure with no dropped eggs or long slow packing. All the shopping was finally in the car, so now the plan was to go home quickly, take everything into the house and put it all away. Simple!

Once inside, P made opening the bag of plums next to impossible, and when I finally managed, the plums flew everywhere. The same thing happened with the apples. My kitchen was beginning to look like a giant fruit salad, and when the mandarins jumped right out of my hand, that was enough. P really was having too much fun with all of this.

Finally everything had been put away, and I took a quick peek at the shopping list that was still there on the table, where I had left it hours ago. I had done better than expected with regards to remembering things I thought to myself as I went down the list. I was impressed and gave P a gleeful smile. Apples - yes, plums - yes, chicken - yes, organic butter… Hang on a minute, organic butter?

Why in heaven's name had I written that down? With a magnifying glass, I took another look at the almost un-readable list. On no, that wasn't organic butter. It was orange bitter, and I had forgotten that. No Queen's Day is complete without orange bitter, it's a tradition.

I was too tired to go to the shops again, so I decided that with all the orange chocolates and pastries no one would miss the orange bitter the next day. I was sure of that, and I was right (luckily).

P&I
Hole in one

The golf club was located on a beautiful lake, surrounded by old trees. It was also the home of many ducks, birds and two lovely swans. They were used to the flying golf balls, but an occasional *squawk* could be heard as a ball failed to reach the grassy area beyond and fell on some unsuspecting duck.

One fine day we left early in the morning. P wouldn't stay alone at home, so we all set off together. When we arrived at the club, he appeared to want to stay in the car. I knew why; it was safer!

It was a perfect day and we decided to take some refreshments on the terrace.

Then it was time to swing a golf club. My husband has always been a fair golfer, I could not claim even the word 'fair', but I could hit the ball OK. First shot, perfect, straight down the line. Second shot, slightly to the left, third shot, *SQUAWK*. Yup, P decided to come out of the car, and a duck had just got a headache. It got worse. Balls were flying in all directions as my co-ordination left me, and I even managed to swing one so far right that it landed on the clubhouse roof. It took the

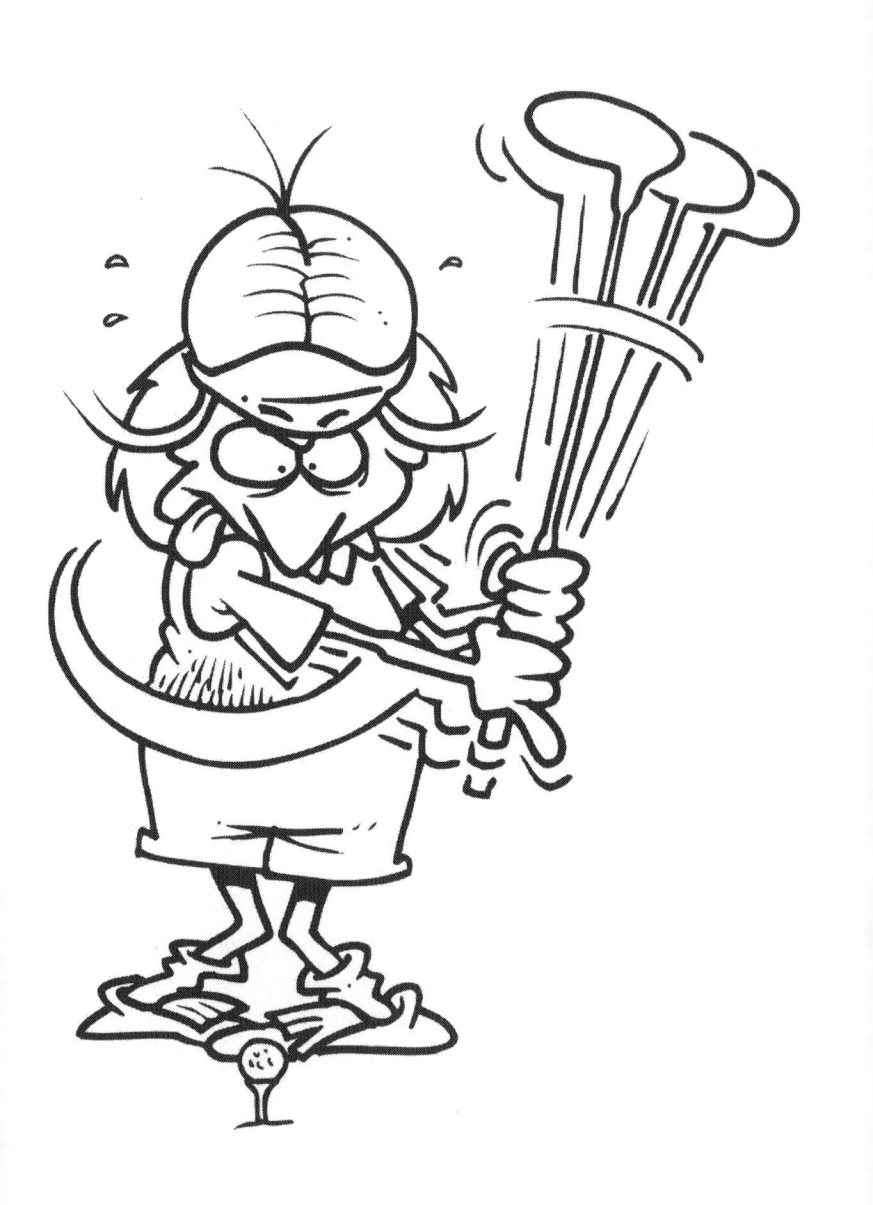

management about five minutes to work out they had a situation on their hands… me!

They arrived ever-so-politely and asked if I was finishing soon. P gave them a little wave and I replied, 'Well not really'. 'Inadequate and unacceptable' was written across their faces, but they said only, 'We don't allow people who are drunk to play on the range, madam.'

Did he say drunk? Never thought of that. P made me appear drunk and I actually found this amusing. I could have said, 'I've got Parkinson's,' but instead opted for, 'Well I only had a few, would you care to join me.' My husband was horrified and the management lost their 'be nice to the drunk lady' look, and said I had to leave.

P was enjoying the confusion, and as I walked off, he sat on my back and made me do that shuffle that I hated so much, but it promoted a softer voice from the managers. 'You cannot even walk straight Madam, I really think you should sit down.'

'No, no I'm used to being in this state all the time,' I replied truthfully. My husband by now was making a beeline for the car grabbing my shoulders on the way.

I wanted to add a hiccup, but thought that was perhaps exaggerating. All in all, P and I had had our fun, and P was not so sulky. My last thought was that, whilst I may have looked drunk, I probably deserved a drink. After all, no harm done – except to the duck!

P&I
The exchange

It was the end of March and there had been frost again during the night. Outside it was horribly cold, but I had to go into town. I needed to exchange a shirt and pick up a book from the bookshop. It was only two shops so it should have been straightforward. Ah! Famous last words.

I had let the dog out and made myself a great cup of hot coffee – it always did the trick of making me feel restored – and I decided to go into town on my bike. P detested the bike and never came with me when I went for a ride.

In the first shop, after explaining that I wanted to swap the shirt I had for a bigger size, the sales lady asked me if it was OK for me to finish the transaction at the other till downstairs. I was laden with shopping and warm clothing, and it was getting hot. Here I was with a too-small shirt in one hand, a bag and a pair of thick gloves in the other. I was wearing my heaviest winter jacket and an enormous scarf – what my husband calls my woolly mammoth look – and as if to make me act like one, P suddenly turned up and began to be a real nuisance. I got a cramp in my right leg and doubled over in pain, the shirt, bag and gloves sent flying.

'Are you alright madam? Would you like to sit down?' Silly question, of course I wasn't alright. I let out a cry of pain.

'Shall I call a doctor?'

'No,' I manage to mutter. 'It's just P!'

'The toilets are over there,' she said pointing to her left.

'Cramp,' I exclaim. 'It's just cramp,' and with tears in my eyes I hobbled downstairs to the other till. As the pain eased, I was able to quickly exchange the shirt and get out of there. Damn P, he loved to spoil my fun.

Outside, the weather had cleared up, and off I was to the bookshop. Once inside, P began to be so annoying that I wanted to give him a good clout. No cramp this time, but a sudden tiredness that had me pinching myself. The pre-ordered book was ready for me to pick up, and, after throwing it into my bag with all my loose change, I dragged myself out of the shop. I slung myself onto my bike, and yearned to be home for my warm lunch. I wondered if anybody has ever fallen asleep riding a bicycle.

At home I gave up being the hero. OK, that day I had won a victory, but not really! When P is involved, every day is a victory. That day I was not going to do any more shopping or run any errands. Cooking was no option either. Fortunately there was a packet of pancake mix in the basement and a carton of ice cream in the freezer. I put the kettle on to make a large pot of tea, and had no doubt that somewhere in the house I could find something nice to eat. I settled myself onto the sofa, sitting in the sun coming in from the window, and trying to enjoy the fact that P had decided to give me a peaceful afternoon. Tomorrow would undoubtedly be the same old story: me getting on with life, and P trying to spoil my fun.

P&I
On the run

On a sunny Sunday afternoon we were driving slowly in our 17-year-old car through the leafy avenues of one of the most beautiful parts of the Netherlands.

It was autumn and we were enjoying the colours of the falling leaves. We approached a picturesque village and decided we would make a stop at the pretty church for a walk. As we entered the village, a police car pulled out and started to follow us. Then came the dreaded flashing lights, and the next moment we were stopped, feeling we had to be very guilty of something, but not sure what. A hunky policeman, looking a bit like Don Johnson, the *Miami Vice* actor, came to the window and my husband greeted him with the habitual, 'Good morning officer! Is there something wrong?'

A scowl, a growl and a curt, 'License and documents please.'

You could see in his face that he was determined that someone should have a bad Sunday. As we were getting out the documents, he walked around the car and looked under it. As if we transported drugs!

'You are in trouble sir,' said the officer with his head

half way through the window. My hair raised up and the metamorphosis went faster than Dr. Jekyll turned into Mr. Hyde. P woke-up and when he saw the police officer he got scared; when P is agitated he makes me stressed. There was a sudden feeling of tension in my body and I knew I needed to move or I would be blocked – which results in not being able to move my leg muscles, a trick P especially enjoyed.

I opened the car door and staggered out. Don looked on incredulously as I started walking a little uncertainly, with my hand shaking up and down beside the car, easing the tension in my body.

'Madam, are you on drugs?' Don asked.

It was a simple question, which could only be answered honestly. 'Well yes quite a few actually.'

Incredulity turned to bafflement as he assessed the situation.

'Please empty your pockets Madam,' so I did. One packet of tissues, one set of keys (ah, I'd wondered where I'd put them), and a large plastic box with pills of various colours.

With triumph in his eyes, Don came nearer. Dreams of promotion for breaking up a major drugs ring were written on his face. A confession, evidence and now the bust, it was in the bag!

I have them in a box divided by hour, so as to remember the right medicine at the right time. I always kept a full 3 days' supply on me for a total of 42 pills.

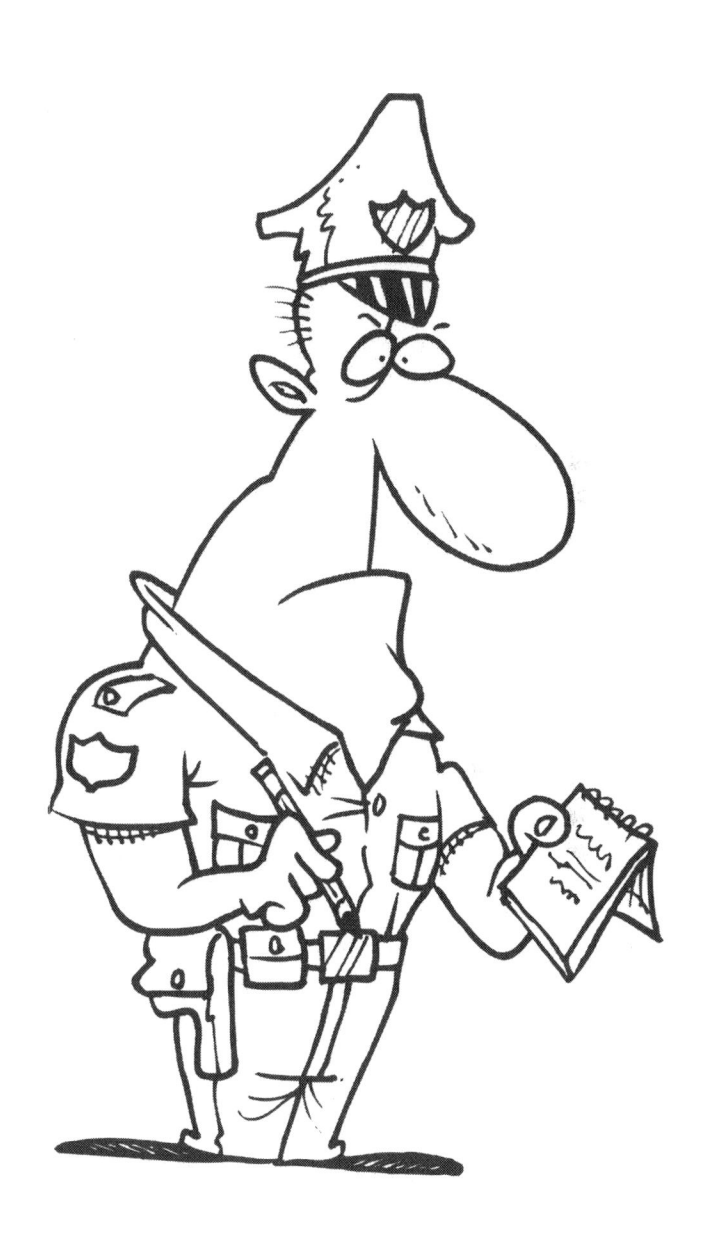

P actually appeared happy, maybe at the thought that the medicines that make him behave better were about to be confiscated. My tension eased and I said casually, 'I have more back at home.'

Don's partner, seeing Don moving in on the suspect, got out of the car, and on analysing the pills said, 'My mother has those big white ones, too.'

Don, not exactly the quickest thinker, stopped in his tracks.

'Have you got Parkinson's, madam?' his partner asked.

'Yes she has,' finally chipped in my husband. Don deflated visibly with his promotion and glory now gone. I then chatted to his partner about P, and eventually got a warm handshake from him, although Don was already back in his car.

Then they were gone. Bizarrely we never got to know what trouble we had been in, unless you count P, who's always a Pain with a capital P.

P&I
The night pharmacy

Friday night around 10 pm I came to the terrible discovery that I had forgotten to pick up my medication. P was ecstatic, especially when I couldn't find the doctor's prescriptions. After some vain attempts searching in coat pockets, kitchen drawers, purses and the complete interior of the car, real panic broke out. Without Levodopa P would have far too much fun at my expense.

Every day, 5 x 125 mg, and I could not miss one! I would never survive P's antics till Monday. There had to be a pharmacy open! If not I'd go to the hospital.

In the car, my husband drove at speed, and I wondered what he would say if the police pulled us over.

'My wife's having a baby,' usually worked, but 'my wife has Parkinson's' probably would get us a ticket. No police this time, and we were soon at the night-pharmacy 20 kilometres away.

The pharmacist, with an air of quiet contemplation, announced, 'I do not have them in stock madam.' He had searched the shelves, but no Levadopa to be found. 'There is some in the vault and that is locked and anyhow is only for emergencies.'

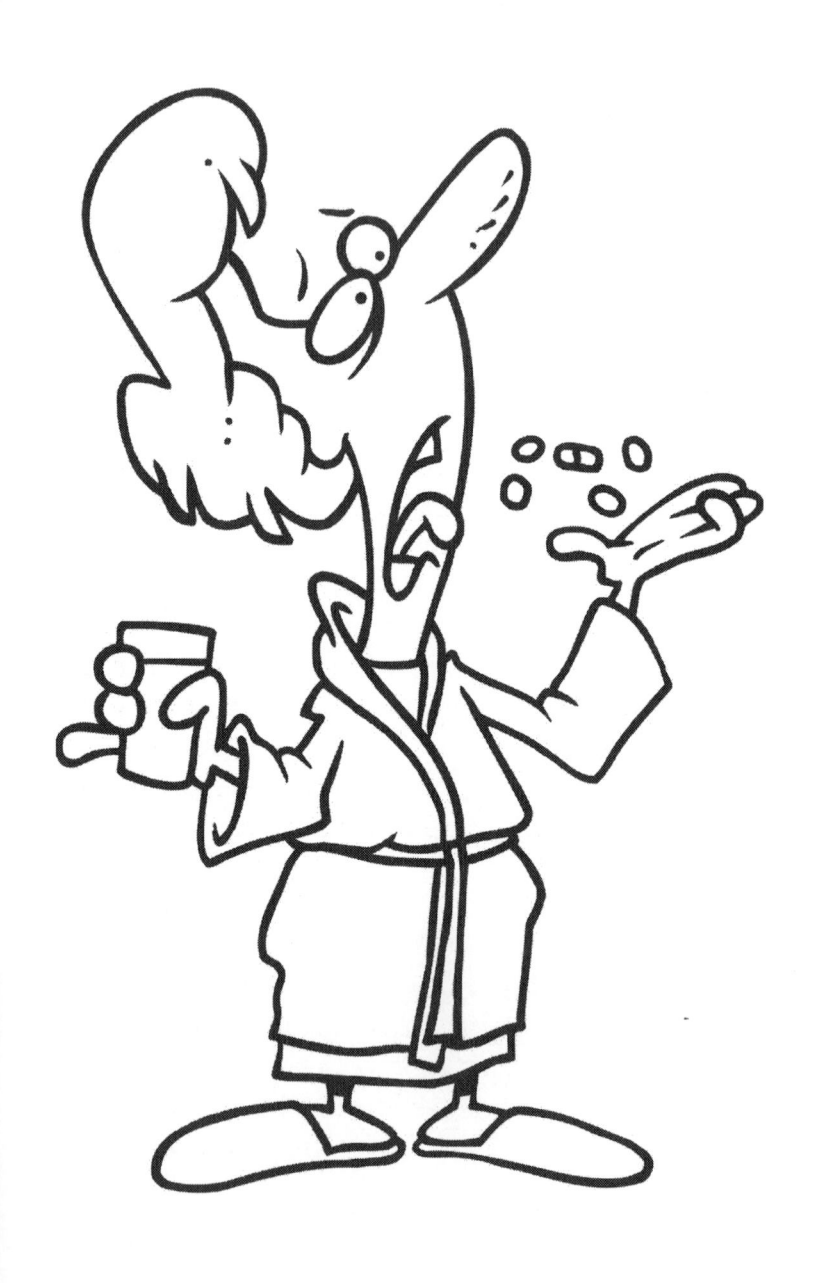

'I am an emergency!' I shouted.

He was not to be moved. 'I dare say you are, but the manager has accidentally taken home the key, and although he lives around the corner, he is staying by the seaside this weekend. So it would take two hours at least before he's here.'

'Help!' Was all that I could think to say.

'I'll deal with the lady behind you, then we can try and call, but you'll need a doctor's prescription.'

Oops, that was a problem. Suddenly, I got a hunch. Fully energised, I snatched the phone out of my bag and tried to call. No signal...

I shuffled outside hoping to get a better reception, whilst running through my contacts for a fellow Parky. A sleepy Jack answered the phone and said he didn't use Sinemet, but suggested I try John. John had been to a party and was half drunk and fully incoherent, so I hung up. But Doreen surely must have Sinemet; I knew that she used it. I phoned her, and yes, she had Sinemet. How much did I need?

Doreen proudly announced she kept a stock as some people are stupid enough to run out. Hmm, subtle hint, but true. We drove to her house and she gave me what I needed. I could have kissed her, but the stiffness that I felt at that point with the lack of medicine made it very challenging.

Taking the pills with a quiet 'thank you,' I knew that with an hour of patience P would be better controlled (and me, too.)

P&I
Yoga lessons

My body was stiff and I could hardly move my arms and legs. I hadn't been to yoga for a long time.

I was feeling resolute, and P must have been still sleeping, so that day I had decided to go to Dolly's studio. Dolly's yoga lessons were more than enjoyable, mainly due to Dolly herself, a tiny 87-year-old lady and agile as a cat. The first hour we talked about making the world a better place and other such improbable discussions: like why men are so stubborn. The second hour we did exercises in which we were frequently astonished by what we could do. The lesson closed with a cup of tea and a plate of delicious organic cookies. We greedily attacked them to a degree where you might think we only came for the cookies.

P always came along at least as far as the front door, where he stayed, just like a wet umbrella. Any further was forbidden territory for him. Sometimes he sneaked in with me but was immediately sent out by Dolly. They detest each other enormously. P didn't like to exercise, and certainly hated yoga.

That day P had stayed with me as I made my way

inside the yoga studio. Dolly didn't want P to disturb the lesson, so she encouraged P to think again about interrupting our precious yoga classes. We progressed with the same improbable discussion, this time about why dogs are more obedient than husbands, and P went to stay with the umbrellas. I forgot P totally, although I knew he was close.

When it was time to go home, it was hard to leave Dolly. She is a very special person. She always has time for other people and makes problems disappear like snow dissolves in the sun.

After that particular lesson, P was not waiting for me with the old umbrellas, but I was sure that he was already at home. I floated home on my old bike, feeling as light and as free as a bird, and completely rid of trembles and aches. Totally relaxed - I wanted to keep this feeling for as long as possible, and today I was going to do so. It took a little time, but I soon realised that I did have control over P if I tried.

P doesn't like exercise, pills, laughter, relaxation or hobbies. Spoilsport, I thought, but I knew that at least I had some control. 'Now how can I apply this to my husband?' I asked myself wistfully. No, husbands were much more complicated,' I reflected. And I saved that thought for our next yoga class discussion.

P&I
The swimming pool

There was a terrible storm outside, as one downpour was followed by another.

We decided that if we were going to get wet we might as well enjoy ourselves doing it, so we headed off to the local covered swimming pool for the first time in years.

You could smell the chlorine as you got to the pool, and all the children inside were doing their best to be heard above the din. The sight of the changing-rooms made me debate whether to turn round and leave at once. P loved chaos, I didn't!

Clad in our multi-coloured costumes, we walked to the edge of the bath. The water should have been 28 degrees but it felt colder. We were here now, so it was just a question of who was going to take the plunge first. I wasn't the first, but when I did enter – more with a splash than a plunge – I realised P had stayed on the poolside edge. No stiff, heavy body, no tired legs, no pain anywhere. I sped through the water like a fish and could dive like a dolphin.

I knew P was afraid of the water, so I tried to tease

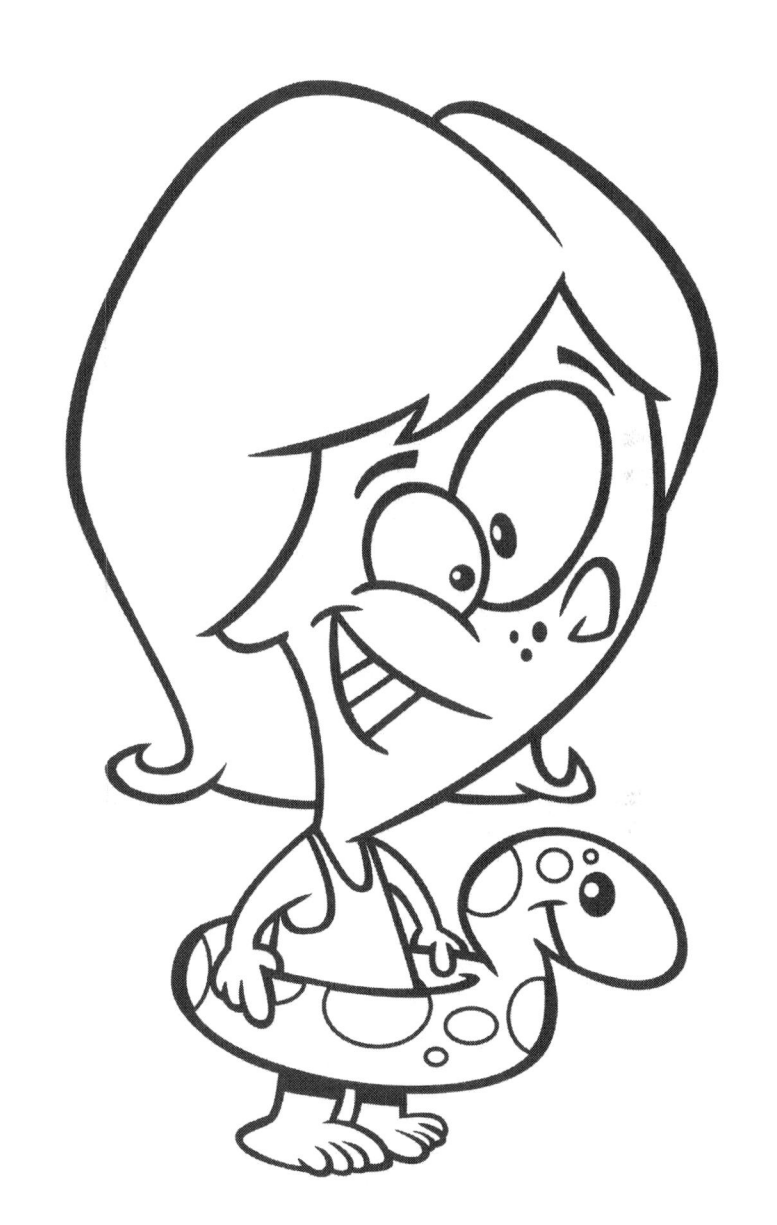

him and enjoyed watching his attempts to follow me. I even suggested we meet in the jacuzzi and raced to the bubbling water. In the bubbles, I felt like a bean in a coffee mill; hidden in a wild cloud of bubbles, I knew no one could see anything of me. It was a strange feeling – as if I was incognito.

With my body feeling like that of a top model, I made an attempt to elegantly climb the smooth pool steps. But it felt like I had sucked all the pool water up the steps with me. As the heaviness returned, I knew P had too. With a bewildered face and hanging on to the steps, I sighed and climbed out. I could lose P sometimes and I could trick him too, but I couldn't shake him off altogether. So P and I walked back to the changing rooms. An odd couple nonetheless.

P&I
The concert

Finally it was almost upon us. The day of the performance approached with rapid steps.

In conjunction with his memorial year, Mozart's *Requiem Mass* was on the programme. After a year of rehearsing, everyone was looking forward to the actual performance.

During the rehearsals it was icy cold in the church, and the singing didn't really get off the ground. To make matters worse, I heard that we had to walk across the stage – first up the steps then over the stage to reach our own chairs – all under the critical eye of our audience. I could feel P planning and contriving for this very moment. I could picture myself, clad in high heels and with my long black dress trailing behind, falling flat on my face.

Heeeeelp!

At eight o' clock on Saturday evening the church was jam-packed full! It was time to take our places, and we followed each other bravely across the stage. The audience applauded and there was no turning back. People had already seen me and P, and sure enough P tried hard to get that spectacular fall I so dreaded, but instead he achieved just a slight wobble and a wave. I smiled. After the performance, my husband said that I had walked strongly across the stage with little sign of P.

I sat there with an impassive face in full view of five hundred people and with my heart pounding in my throat. Panic set in. Okay, here we go, I thought; this was P's playground – stress. I was totally breathless with a trembling hand, trembling leg and shivers inside.

Suddenly, in the right centre of the church, I saw two beloved faces smiling with encouragement. I grabbed P firmly by the collar and pushed him back down. Now it was time to sing, and I sang as never before. P couldn't sing, so sulked moodily.

After we finished, the lady on my left-hand side was visibly emotional. She had enjoyed it. The lady on my right was also moved because it was her last performance. As for me, I was just pleased to have negotiated with P.

P was clearly frustrated, and whilst others filed away, he insisted we stay behind. Blocked, with my legs rooted to the ground and alone on the stage, I felt like a deer in the headlights of a car. P eventually let me go, and I made my way to my husband and daughter, and like the deer that had escaped the headlights, I felt relief rush over me. I'd done it, and P screwed up his face in disapproval.

P&I
The Mexican standoff

The alarm clock rang – it was seven am. Time for my first daily dose of pills. The beeping got irritating, but where was the stupid alarm clock? Not in its usual place. Frantically, I searched for it and discovered it beeping away on the floor beside my bed. In fact, everything was on the floor, including my bedside table, which I must have knocked over.

I looked at the mess next to my bed: pills, tissues, a bottle of hand lotion and a screwdriver. Hmm, how did that get there?

On my knees, I looked under the bed and found my glasses and an empty water cup. P was also awake and seemed to be shouting, 'Yippee, a new day!'

Because I could not take my pills without water, and without pills I could hardly move, I had to go to the bathroom on my hands and knees. Standing up was not an option. And so my husband found me, as he awoke with a yawn, my hair dishevelled, in my nightdress, and on all fours.

I made it to the bathroom, climbed up the sink and filled a cup with water, drinking it together with the pills. I eventually made my way downstairs and opened the curtains, and across the yard I saw the new neighbours doing their gardening. P chose that moment to block my movement. There I was, frozen like an icicle, in my silk nightdress, staring at my new neighbour, who must have thought I was mad, but she waved with a big smile. Then her husband came into view, and I got another wave and big smile. P didn't want to wave back.

It was a Mexican stand-off, with them waving frantically at me, and me rooted to the spot. Who would move first? I'd never been to Mexico, but the stand-off was giving P enormous fun. Too much fun, so I did a shuffle to the right.

I knew I was going to fall before I did the falling, so in panic, I grabbed the curtain and heard the soft sound of ripping fabric. I crumpled to the ground with the curtains on top of me.

My husband, also in his pyjamas, descended the stairs and unwrapped me like a parcel. I could only just mutter, 'Do greet our new neighbours darling.' But by this time the neighbours did not seem to want to greet him and had disappeared from view.

P&I
My dream

In my dream I found myself in a ballroom, where a surprisingly cheerful neurologist, one of a dying breed, was waiting for me. With a firm smack on the shoulder, from which of course I wobbled across the ballroom, he told me that I was one of the lucky ones for whom a cure for Parkinson's would soon be possible.

He gave me an illegible prescription, and referred me to his assistant Flora, who I found, as is the way with dreams, in the toilets.

Flora was an enthusiastic, clearly-enunciating young lady, who reminded me a bit of Lucille Ball. She was singing and holding extra tall flutes of very bubbly champagne. Could you get drunk in a dream? Well I could try!

She asked me to take a seat, which magically appeared by the hand dryer; what a jolly place to be.

Suddenly, we were disturbed by urgent flashing lights. Flora smiled and explained in glee what was going on.

'That is the researchers' alarm. It goes off several times a day. Look!' she said and let me take a peep into the large hall via a monitor.

Hundreds of researchers and professors ran backwards and forwards through the hall as if in panic mode.

'The alarm goes off when they make another discovery, and all the researchers worldwide get the message that we are a step closer to a cure for Parkinson's disease.'

'What happens if they find that something doesn't work?' I mused.

'Ah, that's when the other alarm goes off,' she replied sadly, and as if to prove the point, a toilet flushed behind me.

'Do the lights flash more than the toilet flushes?' I enquired hopefully.

'Oh yes, we get much more flashing than flushing,' she said with a straight face.

So, as I started to wake and Flora faded away, I was left with a positive feeling that, through a flash and a flush, there would be a cure, one day.

Chapter Two
Sally

Sally Bromley

Sally was born in Oxford and still enjoys living there. As a teacher, she always strived to create a stimulating and happy environment for young people to learn in, often encouraging pupils to tell jokes. She also took this humorous approach as an advisory teacher delivering sex education throughout Oxfordshire.

Recently, she has worked in collaboration with others to produce workshops to help people newly diagnosed with Parkinson's to come to terms with the condition. She often gives presentations introducing others to living with Parkinson's.

Her greatest achievement is being a mother and grandmother. Her second greatest achievement was skydiving for charity.

SALLY

The defining moment

I first found out I had Parkinson's when I tried to put a condom on in front of 40 giggling boys.

Oh! I should explain. I was a teacher. In fact I was an advisory teacher – someone who tries really hard to teach those who do not wish to be taught – other teachers. And my chosen subject was sex and relationships education. Yes, I was once described as 'the condom lady.'

I was delivering a lesson on safe sex to 14 year olds; a good age to warn them of the dangers of being promiscuous, even though I feared today's moral values meant in some cases I was a year too late.

I talked about how infections pass from person to person – from nits to HIV. Now I was getting somewhere. So then came the grand demonstration. I got the condom ready, checked it was in date, and carefully opened it and took it out of the package. Immediately, the class started to smirk. Knowing boys well, I understood that half of them thought they knew what I was about to do, but a few had never even seen one before.

Having got the condom out, I unravelled it and held it up. This was looking good. I had the full attention of the class. I looked at their faces and saw gaping mouths, eyes agog and hushed voices. Yeah, I had their attention.

In full view of over 40 boys and a condom in hand, Parkinson's decided to join the show. Parkinson's was in my hand. It took control of my hand... or rather... my hand became totally out of control. The condom was wiggling about. It was shaking, and I suddenly thought of the song *Shake, Rattle and Roll*. But this was no song. It was the moment that I knew I had to see a doctor about my shaking. Meanwhile, Parkinson's had ruined the day.

Some weeks later I saw a neurologist, who, after what seemed no more than a couple of minutes, told me I had early onset Parkinson's. Sadly, because he was busy writing notes I only saw the top of his head as he delivered the news. He didn't even have the courtesy to look me in the eye. I could not resist it; it had to be said and I blurted out, 'I'd hate to be you, having to give such horrid news to people,' and walked out.

After that experience I decided I wanted a second opinion, so I went privately to a clinic in the centre of Oxford to see a young consultant neurologist, who was recommended to me due to her sensitive approach in dealing with people.

I told her about my symptoms and bad sleep. My daughter relayed how I was shouting in my sleep. The consultant asked if there was anything else.

'Err, yes,' I said, and I told her about the shaky condom, adding quickly that I did not see it as funny... She did and smiled.

I also told my work colleagues about the consultation and my condom calamity. One of my colleague's wives told me how much she enjoyed the story and that whenever she feels down or miserable, she thinks of me with my hand holding the condom and Parkinson's doing his thing in front of 40 boys. It greatly cheers her up, apparently.

And so Parkinson's entered my life.

Let's go out for lunch

A mid-week lunch with a fellow Parky sounds simple, right? A pub meal beside the gentle flowing waters of the river. Idyllic.

The menu looked good and we started working out which meals we could eat. You see, Parkinson's often stops the hand from doing what you want it to do, and cutting things on a slippery plate is one such thing. Our meals arrived and my friend got stuck into hers. I looked at my plate and shivered with fear. I had ordered ribbon vegetables, but they were not as I had imagined. I guess I thought it would be more like a coleslaw. But no, these vegetables were worthy of a best-in-show award. They were huge and very long.

I tried cutting them to no avail. I tried using my fingers, but that didn't work either as they were slippery with dressing, and one carrot shot across the room, narrowly missing the desert trolley. It dawned on me that even if I eventually got them to my mouth, I'd look a bit like Lassie the dog with a bone. Not attractive!

This called for some serious cutting. But who? No staff visible. Everyone around us: eating with friends. Me: unable to get food to my mouth. Ah, just behind me were two men. Two young men. In fact, two young and good looking men. Yes, I'd target them.

'Excuse me,' I said. They looked my way, and I nearly lost my nerve.

'Excuse me, but could you cut my vegetables up for me?'

They were astonished and a little confused, but one kindly moved up close and cut the ribbons up for me.

I am quite sure that neurologists should add a new test for Parkinson's. The 'spaghetti test' would be far more accurate than many that are used today.

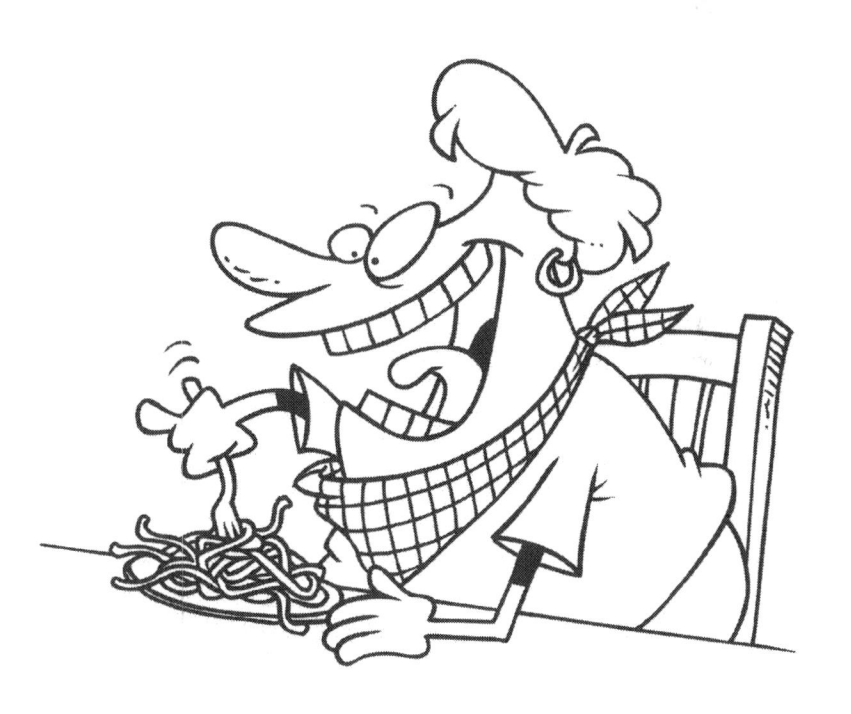

Eating spaghetti is difficult for many people, but it is particularly so for anyone with Parkinson's. On a recent trip to Italy, we went to a restaurant where I ordered the famous Italian dish, and when it arrived I stuck the fork in and twirled... or rather I told my hand to twirl. But the message never reached my hand. I looked at my husband with a helpless look of distress. He understood, phew. He reached over and twirled my spaghetti – mouthful by mouthful – for me.

And the next day, guess what was the first course at the hotel? Yes you guessed it right. *Primo* was spaghetti again. 'No', I whispered to my husband. 'No, I am not going to give up today.'

I cut up the spaghetti, asked for a spoon and scooped it up – a cardinal sin in Italy, as I discovered later - but nobody said a word.

On my return to the UK, I was being interviewed for research by a charming Italian doctor. I proudly told him of my visit to Sicily and said I'd found a perfect way to diagnose Parkinson's. 'I reckon the ability to twizzle spaghetti onto a fork would be a simple way to diagnose if someone has Parkinson's,' I said.

He looked serious when he asked what I meant. I described my first meal at the restaurant when my husband twirled spaghetti on my fork.

His face dropped.

'He put it on your fork?' he said with incredulity. I nodded and explained my second meal, which I'd cut up myself. A look resembling *The Scream* by Munch came over his face. Then he covered his face with his hands and shook his head. When eventually he raised his face up to me, he showed no interest in my newly-found diagnostic, but did explain most eloquently how getting someone to twirl spaghetti onto your fork, and worse still to cut it all up, is really not acceptable. Needless to say, I never saw him again.

Chapter Three
Richard

Richard Tyner

Richard is the firstborn of nine children, which has stood him in good stead throughout his career.

In 1967, his family emigrated from Ireland to Peterborough, UK. He has worked for Shell UK Oil, EMAP and Lloyds TSB, but by far and away his most important work has been as a presenter of the *First Steps* programme for the Parkinson's newly diagnosed.

His greatest individual moment was as a Games Maker at the 2012 Olympics.

His greatest family moments were the birth of his two daughters, and watching them receive their degrees in biology and chemistry.

RICHARD

A sock changed my life

I learnt to live with Parkinson's thanks to a sock!

Some years ago now, having just started my career, I was bumped up to management level, much to my surprise and everybody else's, too.

Now, never having had the responsibility of running a department, I was unschooled in the ways of diplomacy and tact. My idea of tactful was to shout, but not quite as loudly as normal. If someone wanted me to do something at work then I did it; I guess it must be my Irish roots. I was born with a natural acceptance of authority and an inclination to go out of the way in order to please others. All this did not bode well for my newly-elevated status, and indeed at first I was both confused and scared.

I overestimated my power to make people do something and underestimated the British habit of questioning orders. I was in control, but with no control, and chaos soon ensued.

I knew that some people were unhappy with my promotion and in particular, the wife of the guy who did not get my job was waiting for me to make a mistake, and I was, in the end, surprised she had to wait so long. My first six months as a supervisor were sheer hell.

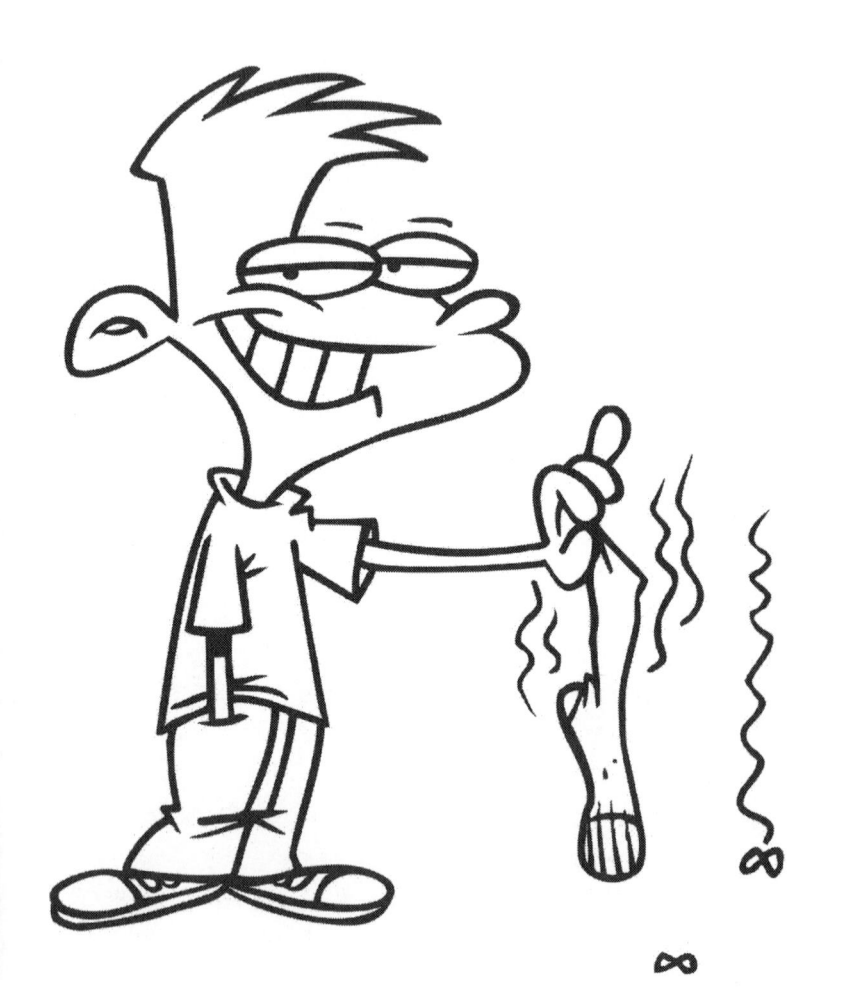

RICHARD

I often found not only that my orders were ignored, but actually being misread on purpose. I once asked a bloke to get the stock checked, only to get the reply four hours later that the stock was still there. 'Count the stock!' I tactfully shouted, to which he replied, 'But that'll take all day and it's home time in five.'

I guess nobody had the heart or guts to tell me that I was not in control and a bossy boss, until one day I remember receiving a padded envelope addressed to 'Richard Tyner, Data Controller'. Inside the envelope was a single black sock. Surprise turned to disbelief, as attached to it were the words *Put a sock in it mate*. I got the point, and the next day came to work with two black shoes and one black sock. The joke was on me... literally, and it soon became clear that I had changed my ways.

So what has this got to do with my Parkinson's? Well put simply, I learnt to listen, I learnt to be sensitive to other people's problems and feelings, which led me to take on the role as chair of my local Parkinson's branch. I worked hard to make the lives of the members more fun, and help take their minds off their condition. The two years I stayed as chair were amongst the most fulfilling of my life, and to think, if it had not been for a sock in the post I may never have learned the skill of how to treat people properly.

P.S. I still have that sock.

Mum's the word

By way of preparation for life, being the eldest of nine is up there amongst the best of them. 'Preparation' is perhaps the wrong word for being diagnosed with Parkinson's though.

I knew there was a problem, but when my wife finally said, 'You walk like a penguin, talk quietly and are stiff as a board. I think you should make an appointment with the doctor,' I booked the appointment immediately.

Three weeks later I had been passed up the line and found myself with an appointment at a neurological clinic. The various scenarios ran through my mind: brain tumour, MS, MSA, Alzheimer's? Modern technology is so advanced, and given the costs of the tests I'd expected at least a bright, shiny technical marvel to produce the answer. I was wrong. There I was, made to click my fingers, stamp my feet and be pushed violently from behind by a neurologist with medical degrees and years of experience in finger clicking and the gentle art of shoving people.

'Yes you have got Parkinson's.' I held my breath for a more detailed and insightful explanation of his diagnosis, but instead I got some booklets and a pack of pills.

I found over the following weeks that a neurologist was perhaps not the best person to explain life after diagnosis: the translation of finger clicking into diagnosis – yes, but life afterwards – no.

I found that it was my mother who proved the best preparation for what was to come. Well, more precisely, her words and common sayings like, 'When we fall down, get up again' or, 'When a door closes, open another one', or again, 'When all is said and done, there is a lot more said than done'.

She taught me many other lessons in life, including the survival of the fittest and that effort reaps rewards. I have to add that many of my mother's phrases were hard to understand, and I spent much of my childhood trying to work out their meaning. We used to laugh when she told us each separately and privately that we were her favourite. It did not take us long to work out that she had nine favourites. One of her more insightful comments was that an argument was an exchange of ignorance, whilst a discussion was an exchange of intelligence.

She taught us to stand on our own two feet, knowing that one day we would take the emigrant boat to England or the USA. Don't chase money, chase success, she'd say, insisting that money is a by-product of success and that it was important for us to dream.

I accepted my diagnosis more easily than most thanks to my mother, and I made my mind up that I was going to live each day like there is no tomorrow. That was March 2007. Today I find that my neurologist continues to shove me in the back and still mutters 'interesting' every time he does so. I'm glad he finds such interest from such a minor thing; for me every day is interesting, because you never know quite what it will bring.

Chapter Four
John

John Foster

John is a children's writer who has edited over 100 anthologies of poetry for children, including the best-selling Twinkle Twinkle Chocolate Bar. He has written 12 books of his own poetry and has visited over 500 schools and performed his poems at the Edinburgh and Cheltenham festivals. He is well-known for his performances as a rapping granny and dancing dinosaur.

He taught for over 20 years, before becoming a full-time writer, and is also the author of many educational textbooks and books for teachers, such as the *Your Life* series of personal, social and health education books, which have sold over a million copies.

John was diagnosed with Parkinson's at the age of 64. He has had DBS (deep brain stimulation), an operation that puts electrodes into the brain to moderate the tremor and other symptoms.

JOHN

Driving through the airport

I was offered Deep Brain Stimulation five years after I was diagnosed with Parkinson's. This is basically a simple operation that electrocutes my brain into behaving – well it stimulates it to work!

The tremor in my right arm at the time was getting progressively worse, so I decided to go ahead with the operation. Having the tremor controlled would make me less anxious about doing things socially. Indeed, it made it possible to do many things that were becoming difficult, for example to play chess with my grandson without knocking over the pieces whenever it was my move. Unfortunately, it would not help me win, but at least I could lose with style!

My grandson was fascinated by the remote control I was given, and was keen to experiment with turning the battery on and off.

'You're remote controlled,' he said. 'Show me how it works!'

'It's not a toy,' I said. 'It's to help me get the right setting to control the tremor, and to check that I haven't done anything to damage the stimulation that I'm receiving. And I've got to avoid anything magnetic that might interfere with the battery.'

'You mean like the security gates they have at airports?' he asked. He thought about it for a moment. 'What would happen if you went through one? Would the battery explode?'

'No,' I said laughing. 'But it might create enough interference to turn the battery off, to interfere with the setting or to give me an uncomfortable feeling in my arm.'

I recalled this conversation as my wife and I arrived at Birmingham airport on our way to a holiday in Fuerteventura, one of the Canary Islands. I'm not a very good passenger at airports. I always get anxious that we'll lose our boarding passes or arrive at the gate after it has been closed.

So I approached airport security anxiously. The doctors had told me to present the card they had given me to the guard and ask them to frisk me instead of making me go through the security arch.

These days you have to take off your belt and shoes, which are difficult for someone with Parkinson's, and put them in the tray to go through the scanner. So I had to stand by the arch waving the card with one hand and trying to hold my trousers up with the other, and all the time making sure the guard didn't get anywhere near me with his magnetic wand.

At Birmingham airport, everything went smoothly and I went through security without incident. It was at security at Fuerteventura, on the way back, that things nearly went awry. I presented the card, which the guard took and examined. He looked puzzled and turned it over, where there is an explanation in five languages that I have an implanted medical device that may set off an airport security system. One of the languages is Spanish, and I assumed he would read that and understand.

But he handed back the card, still looking a bit puzzled.

'You have a pacemaker?' he asked.

'No,' I said. 'I have a battery. For Parkinson's.'

He clearly didn't understand. I wondered what he would do.

He looked at me for a moment, then asked me to hold out my arms as he frisked me, then waved me through. I heaved a sigh of relief.

My wife found me a seat and left me putting on my shoes as she went in search of a coffee shop. I put my shoes back on and took out the card to put it back into my wallet. As I did so, I looked at it and immediately began to laugh. For the card I had presented to the guard wasn't the one about the implanted battery, but my UK driving licence!

A routine ECG

You may think that having an ECG is just a routine procedure that most people will experience either when they go for a health check or into hospital for an operation. Well, it is for the majority of patients, but not for those who have Parkinson's and have a tremor. Routine becomes farce in that case.

'Just keep still,' says the nurse operating the machine.

'Well, I would if I could,' is my honest reply, but it falls on deaf ears as the nurse looks at the printout, then crumples it up with a tut-tutting sound.

'I won't be a moment,' she says and goes out of the room. She returns with another nurse.

'We'll try again,' she says. 'My colleague will hold your arm and help you to keep still.'

This was getting interesting. Perhaps this could be a new therapy for stopping arm tremor.

So she gets the machine ready.

'OK. We're ready,' she says.

Her colleague grips my hand and we are locked together, but still the shaking continues as another graph is drawn.

The nurse looks at it and sighs, then crumples it up.

'One more go,' she says. Her colleague grips me

more firmly. She is a large lady, but her arm lock fails once again as Parkinson's continues to move my hand like an invisible force.

The nurse looks at the printout. 'That'll have to do,' she says, shaking her head, which I interpret as 'I give up!'

I thought it would be easier when I'd had the DBS implant, but it proved difficult for a different reason. The battery interfered with the ECG machine, producing graphs that were difficult to decipher.

The health care assistant was getting so exasperated that I offered to switch the system off to enable her to get a reading. She looked taken aback. 'I'm not agreeing to that. I'm not taking responsibility,' she said.

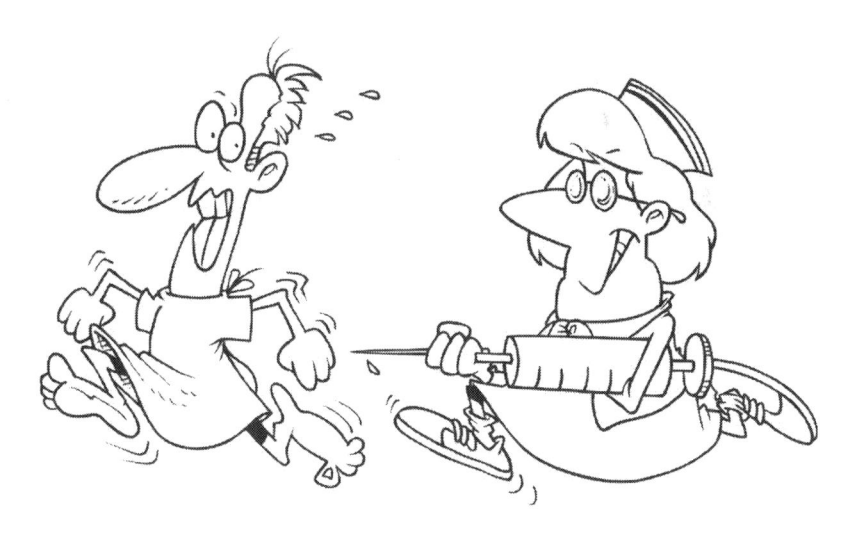

'It'll be all right. My wife and I know how to operate it,' I said, reversing roles, as I, the patient, tried to reassure the health care assistant.

'He can grip the side of the bed,' said my wife.' And then I'll switch him back on.' Making me sound like a washing machine

But the assistant wasn't convinced and made full haste to the nearest doctor.

My wife and I started to giggle. 'She's twitched,' I said. 'It's shaken her confidence.'

We straightened our faces as she re-entered the room. 'The duty doctor says I've got to get on with it, so we'll go ahead,' she said. 'But I'm not at all happy about this.'

But with my wife in charge of the DBS control unit, and me clutching the side of the bed tightly we succeeded in getting a readable printout.

'I knew that would work,' she said with a gleeful expression. We just smiled.

To tell or not to tell

One of the most difficult things about having a tremor is whether or not to explain to everyone you come into contact with that it's because you have Parkinson's. You are introduced to someone and they want to shake your hand, which shakes in turn as you hold it out. To tell or not to tell, that is the question.

People's reactions are very different, ranging from, 'I thought it might be Parkinson's' to, 'Oh, I'm so glad that's the reason, I thought it was because you were an alcoholic.' Then there was the plumber who jumped to conclusions and said he was sorry I'd had a stroke. Perhaps most bizarre of all was the remark made by someone I met at a party. He was clearly interested in how the tremor affected all aspects of my life for he said, 'I suppose you must be careful when you have a pee otherwise you'll shake it everywhere.'

Adults are more self-conscious about how to react than children, who just accept that you've got a shaky arm and are curious to know why. When I visited schools to perform my poems, before I had DBS, I would explain to the children that I had a condition called Parkinson's and that my arm shook. I'd ask them to ignore it and listen to the words, and most of them would do so. Often, one of the pupils would come up to me afterwards to tell me that a relative or friend of their family had Parkinson's too.

A member of staff in one school said what a good role model I was. I thought this was taking things a bit far, until she explained that there was a child in her class with a tremor. She introduced me to him. We shook together and he chortled with glee.

Nowadays, thanks to DBS, I can do a performance in a school without any of the children realizing that there's anything wrong. Running poetry workshops isn't quite so easy, though. I get the children to make suggestions and write them on the board, but the squiggles I make bear little resemblance to the words they suggest.

The DBS controls the tremor, but my handwriting continues to deteriorate. I still draft my poems by hand. 'Can you read what you write?' people sometimes ask me, as they struggle to decipher what I've written. 'No,' I reply. 'Can you?'

Using the computer is frustrating, too. I tend to hit two keys rather than one and I am constantly having to remove typos. I've come up with some amusing ones, though. I recently wrote the title of a book I'm currently working on as 'Brilliant Ideas for

Peaking and Lustening'!

Fortunately, my voice isn't affected when I give talks, but I have to be careful not to stumble over the words of my rapping granny piece, as granny disappears into the distance rapping away to her heart's content!

Chapter Five
Paul

Paul Mayhew-Archer

Paul taught for three years. He organized one school trip and got left behind.
Then in 1979 he joined the BBC comedy department and has worked in comedy ever since.
He co-wrote *The Vicar of Dibley* and more recently worked on *Mrs. Brown's Boys*.
He also co-wrote *Roald Dahl's Esio Trot*, starring Dustin Hoffman and Judi Dench, and is now writing a comedy about Parkinson's. In 2016 he ventured into factual television and presented a BBC 1 documentary called *Parkinson's: The Funny Side*.
'My father was married to my wife's mother, which means I am married to my step sister and I am my son's uncle. With a background like that it's hard to take anything seriously.'

Diagnosis...
they say the strangest things

Five years ago I was telling a friend about my tiny handwriting, and the way my arm didn't swing when I walked, and he said:

'I don't want to worry you, Paul, but those are the symptoms my father had when he was diagnosed with Parkinson's.'

I resisted the temptation to ask my friend what he said when he DID want to worry someone, and I went to see a neurologist.

The neurologist watched me walk up and down his office, he prodded me in the chest, he prodded me in the back, and then he said:

'Yes that's Parkinson's.'

My wife asked, 'You can tell? From just that?'

'Well no,' he said. 'Also your facial muscles are quite frozen. For instance you seem to find it quite difficult to smile.'

'That could be because you've just told me I have Parkinson's,' I said.

Since then I've discovered that we all have our individual diagnosis stories.

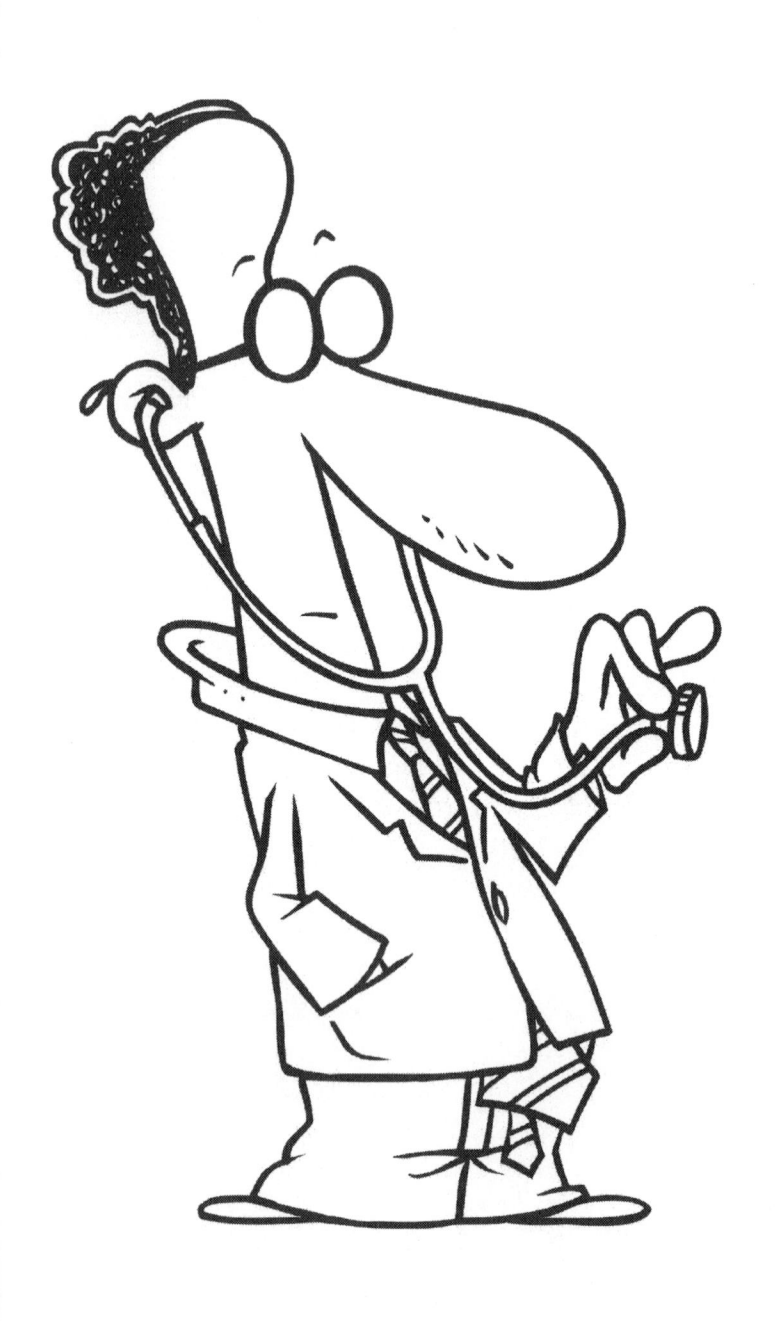

PAUL

There was the neurologist who told a patient, 'You could suffer any number of symptoms, from losing your voice to losing your memory. The only things we know are that it is incurable and it will get progressively worse.'

And then he added helpfully, 'But don't look it up on the internet because that'll just depress you.'

My favourite though is the neurologist who liked treating his patients to a rollercoaster ride of emotions as he delivered information.

'You should expect five good years,' he told one patient at their first meeting. 'Having said that, there is absolutely no reason why you should be in a wheelchair when you're seventy-five.'

'Phew. That's a –'

'But you might. We don't know.'

A year later the same patient asked the same neurologist whether Parkinson's affected life expectancy. And the neurologist said, 'That's a very interesting question because we used to think it did affect life expectancy, but then about six years ago we decided that it didn't.'

'Phew. That's a –'

'But now we think it does.'

Mind you, it isn't only neurologists who say the wrong thing. I met a man in my hometown and he asked, 'How are you?' in a tone of voice that suggested he thought I didn't have long to live.

'I'm well,' I said cheerily. 'I've been having a good laugh working on a comedy show.'

'Oh, that is good,' he said. 'It's good to laugh while you still can.'

Actually that is a phrase I've encountered more than once. A charity worker said to me, 'We want to use you in a forthcoming fundraising event. We want to get the most out of you while we still can.'

So finally, what's the most inappropriate thing anyone has said to someone with Parkinson's?

Well it was said by *me*. I met someone a few months ago and I immediately recognised the tell-tale signs of the arm not swinging and the frozen facial muscles. I introduced myself, explained that I also had Parkinson's and asked him when he'd been diagnosed.

'I haven't been,' he said.

Finding the positives

Two years ago I became chair of governors at a local primary school. They were looking for a volunteer and my arm shot up. It was a Parkinson's twitch, but I was elected nonetheless.

I have really enjoyed the role and I would never have done it without Parkinson's.

Of course, Parkinson's also makes life difficult for me, but sometimes those difficulties can lead to a funny story.

A couple of years ago I was asked to judge a local talent show in our town square. I was also asked if the local radio station could do a phone interview with me just before the contest.

'Fine,' I said. 'Call me ten minutes before it begins.'

I got to the square twenty minutes before the event and waited for the call, and that is when I felt the urge to have a pee.

Now, as anyone with Parkinson's knows, you can be fine one second, then feel you've got to go the next. So, without hesitation, I ran to the loos in the Guildhall.

Two other things anyone with Parkinson's will know are that a) you pee sitting down, and b) you don't take your coat off because you'll be hours getting it back on again.

So there I was, sitting on the loo, hitching my coat up behind me, shifting myself forward so I could properly hitch it up, shifting myself forward a little bit more and then finding I've shifted myself so far forward I am peeing straight into my trousers.

And that was when the phone rang.

I can't say it was the best interview I've ever given. It's hard to focus your thoughts when the interviewer asks if you can 'Do something about the echo,' and when a lavatory attendant bangs on your door, shouting, 'Who are you talking to? We don't allow couples in there.'

And then I had to go straight out and judge the talent contest.

A couple of months later I told this story at a quiz evening I was running, and a woman came up and thanked me.

'I was diagnosed with Parkinson's two weeks ago,' she said. 'And I felt as though my life was over. But seeing you with the disease and still able to laugh about it - well - I don't feel so bad now.'

So let's all look for the positives in Parkinson's – the new friendships we will make, the opportunities it will present, and the laughs it will give us.

Memories of therapy (at the European Parkinson Therapy Centre)

I had the pleasure of spending a week at the European Centre in Italy, with none other than Sally Bromley, another Parky who was with me for the week.

At the start of the week we were both given pedometers, and every day I was proud to announce I had completed 10,000 steps – then dismayed to discover that Sally was doing at least 3,000 more.

'Well done Sally,' everyone would say. 'You must do better Paul. Why can't you do as many steps as Sally?'

'Because she takes smaller steps! She's a girl,' I would shout pathetically. But it was no use. Sally was the gold medallist and I was the hopeless Brit who trailed in last.

Then – in a revelation to equal the discovery of the Russian Federation's systematic cheating at the London Olympics – we discovered the sordid truth. Sally Bromley, golden girl, put her pedometer in her dressing gown pocket every morning. And Sally Bromley, pedometer princess, has shaky leg syndrome, so she was doing 2000 steps over breakfast.

SHAKEN BUT NOT STIRRED

The Parkinson Centre is in a spa town called Boario Terme. I'm now 62 and I loved the relaxed atmosphere of the place where nobody jogged and everyone strolled, and afternoon tea dances took place in the park.

Also – this being Italy – there was always a very elderly Catholic nun sitting in the hotel lobby. Was she a real nun, we wondered, or a prop?

And the hotel was conveniently close to the Therapy Centre. A gentle stroll of 200 steps – or if you're Sally Bromley, 400 steps.

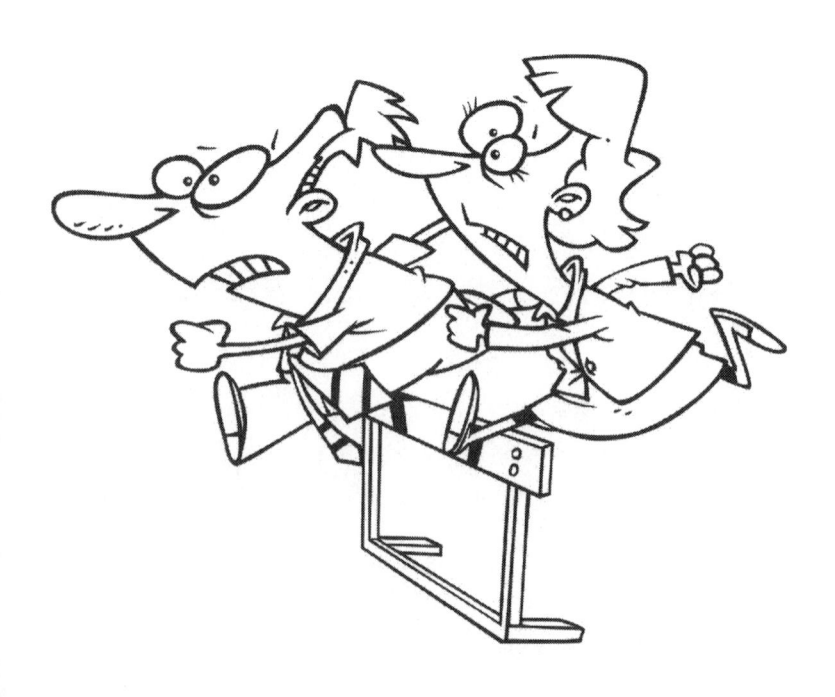

PAUL

Then, once I entered the therapy centre there was no more strolling, there was no more enjoyment of the relaxed atmosphere, there was Agata.

Agata, the 25 year old, tiny pocket tyrant who would order me to run, run faster, run even faster, walk sideways on the treadmill (you try walking sideways on a treadmill!!), pedal harder on the exercise bike and put more power into my power exercises. For ninety minutes every morning she would make me work like I have never worked in my life. And I loved her for it.

One therapy I did enjoy was to go to the ice cream shop opposite the hotel, order a cone and ask for a squirt of liquid chocolate. Then a scoop of chocolate ice cream. Then cream. Then another squirt of liquid chocolate. Oh, yes.

The centre is run by Alex who is the architect of the program Agata was so enthusiastically applying. There is a simple reason why the program works as well as it does, and why it made me feel so much better and more in control of my condition. Alex has many qualities as a designer and manager, but he has something more important – he has Parkinson's.

Then came the moment....

We ended a session on handwriting with some breathing exercises. We all closed our eyes and breathed in… and breathed out.

There was a very elderly Italian man on the course who could barely move. Every time he breathed out he suddenly started moaning. It was such a loud and distinctive moan that Sally and I could not help but open our eyes and give each other a 'isn't-that-the-weirdest-moan-you've-ever-heard' look. Then when he moaned again I'm afraid we giggled.

The man then whispered to his wife in Italian, and she smiled and translated, 'My husband says he is moaning because he is dreaming of cake.'

And we all laughed. And then he laughed. And then she cried a little because it had been a long time since she had heard him laugh.

That simple moment – a man hardly able to move, laughter and tears – that's Parkinson's.

Chapter Six
Alex

Alexander Reed

Alex was born in Uganda, raised in the UK and lives in Italy. All very confusing, but logical, as he is married to an Italian with two children.

After various directorships, Alex became a consultant before being diagnosed at age 46.

With support from USA, UK and Italy, he opened and is the director of the non-profit European Parkinson Therapy Centre, which has become a leading centre for early stage Parkinson's.

His biggest success was learning Italian and then persuading one to marry him.

His dream is to transfer care services for Parkinson's into a multilevel support system, turning people with Parkinson's into protagonists, not patients.

His stories are taken from his experiences working as a volunteer at the Centre.

The slippery slope

I first met Gio on a Sunday; he was alone yet appeared at ease with himself. A remarkably funny man, although very hard to understand at times with his full-blown Naples accent.

'So how do I get rid of Parkinson?' were his first words. Well I thought that was what he said, as with his accent it could have equally been 'How do I get fed and some party fun?'

Not knowing which it was, I played safe and said, 'You can't.' This appeared to be accepted, but he went on to say more clearly, 'Parkinson's interferes with my life'.

Well yes it would, and I gave the standard 'take control' speech and left it at that.

A couple of days later I started to get a clearer picture of what he meant.

'I live with my family but we argue all the time,' he remised. I was not surprised at this, as I had already discovered that his wife knew about his 'other woman', and it appeared that the 'other woman' was not that pleased either.

'Women,' he declared. 'You can't live with them, but I can't live without them.'

'Indeed,' I replied. 'But you don't live with the one you can't do without.'

This appeared to surprise him and he expressed his strong allegiance to his family.

Italians, I thought, have a logic unknown to mere mortal man.

His children had taken their mum's side but stayed on speaking terms. I interpreted this as being because Gio had a large bank account and a 'strong allegiance' to his family, translated as being he was generous to a fault.

His Parkinson's was not that advanced, and he responded well to treatment. But as further revelations were made about his chaotic social life it became clear that, to use a metaphor, even though his Parkinson's was mild, when you live full speed with a wobbly wheel, you are going to get shaken up and have difficulty staying on the road. I then discovered that not only did he have a wheel problem, but his whole life was seriously in danger of falling apart. As he recounted, 'I've got 3 businesses and two are heavily in debt. In short I'm a duck.' Given his accent, he may well have meant a word similar to 'duck' but with a more emphatic meaning.

We waved goodbye with promises of staying in close contact, and to my surprise we did. His calls showed he was sinking deeper into debt and despair. His children were demanding even more 'allegiance', and his Parkinson's was showing signs of being more than an

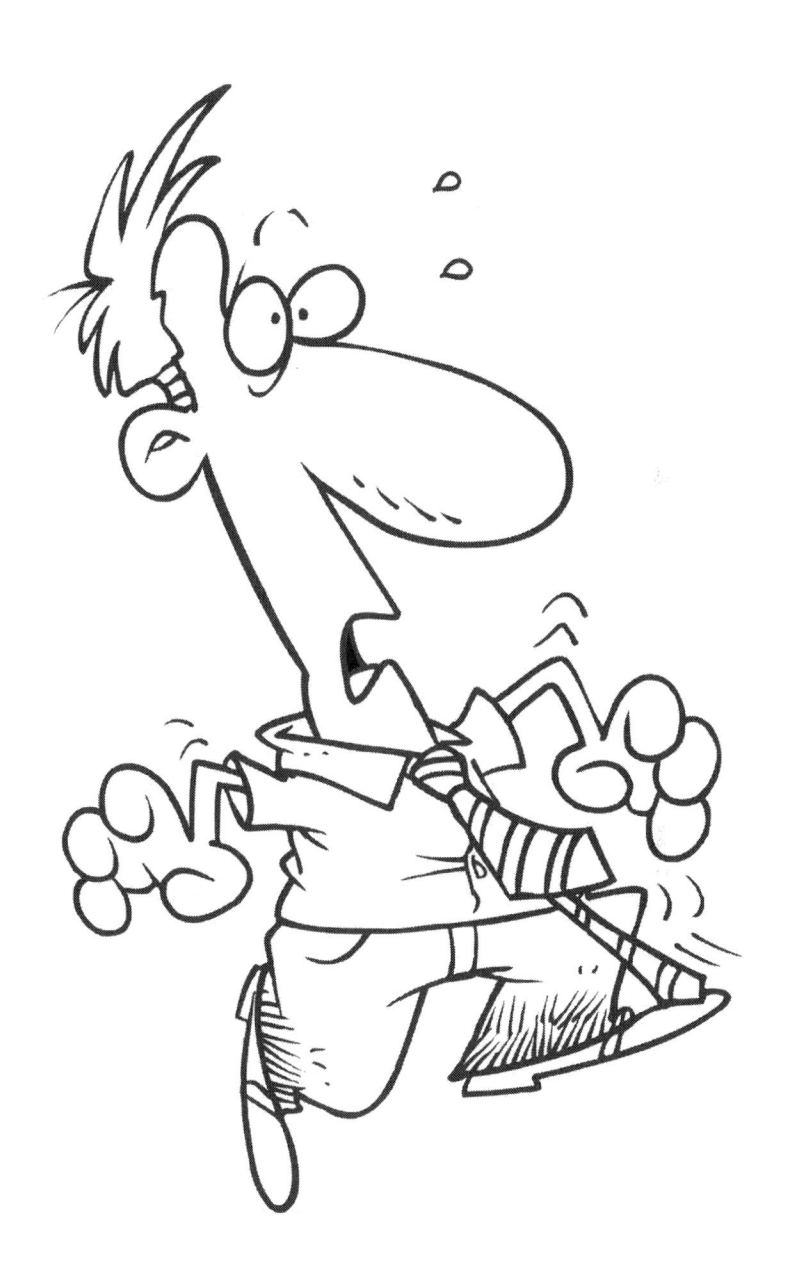

interference to his life. I'd seen this happen many times before, full speed living with a Parkinson's car.

Eventually, I got him into a hospital where he was 'checked over' – medically speaking – with a resultant increase of medicines.

'I grew a hand' he said to me, which by now I could understand as meaning, 'I'm a new man.'

Well, he was then, but it didn't last long, and the next time I spoke to him he had a medical dopamine drip. His Parkinson's did not call for such a radical medical approach and I told him in clear words 'GET CONTROL or you are indeed a duck!'

He made the usual promises and a long speech about friends and gratitude, but I did not get my hopes up.

I was wrong! His next call one month later was to announce that he was coming to see me for a celebratory lunch. Two days later he rolled into town in his Lexus, driven by a driver, and embraced me like I was his long-lost brother. The driver obviously didn't have a brother as he just nodded a greeting. 'I've got rid of that damn drip,' he announced. 'And I've got my medicines down to 4 a day minimum dose.'

I was intrigued, and as he saw my puzzled face he threw his arms around me again. This was beginning to get uncomfortable, especially when he said, 'You are more than a friend'. Looking for an interpretation of his behaviour, I asked what had happened since we last met. Ah, just the opening he had been waiting for, and in rapid excited Italian he rattled off the answer.

'I moved out from the house, dumped the girlfriend, closed the two companies and moved in with my driver. I'm relaxed and feeling good, you must come down and stay; it has been so erotic!' I hoped he meant 'chaotic', but couldn't be sure, so I detached myself from his grasp and smiled.

'So, you took control then? And you slowed down and took away stress?'

He looked at me, and I knew I was about to get another exuberant embrace, and he said with a sly smile, 'I'm not a duck anymore!'

A strange case of blocking

Of all the people I've met, she was the most fascinating. A grandmother with tussled hair and a wit that never failed to surprise me.

'Don't worry about me dear, I'm not running away,' she said shuffling in the direction of the main hall. 'I'm just going to get changed,' she told me once. Half an hour later and with no sign of my favourite grandmother, I went to investigate and found her blocked (freezing of muscles may occur in some people with Parkinson's) in the changing room. We tried all the usual techniques, and even resorted to an outburst of 'That's the Way I Like it', as rhythm sometimes helps in such occasions, although our lack of singing ability may have undermined our efforts. It somehow partially worked, as she heartedly joined in on the chorus, but still no movement.

It took us three days and many more song titles to work out that she blocked almost at will, through anxiety or self-conviction. Whilst our singing improved, she did not. She hated her routine to be broken, and just like a child would throw a tantrum; she would block and there she would remain, still singing along to the chorus-lines but not moving.

ALEX

On the last day, we needed to convince her that her blocking was caused partly by self-conviction and stress. So we unexpectedly changed the time of an appointment, added that she needed to stay through lunch for some tests, and watched as she became agitated, and then went rigid as she found herself blocked again. If she could convince herself to block, she could convince herself to move, with or without our rendition of 'Hit Me Baby One More Time'.

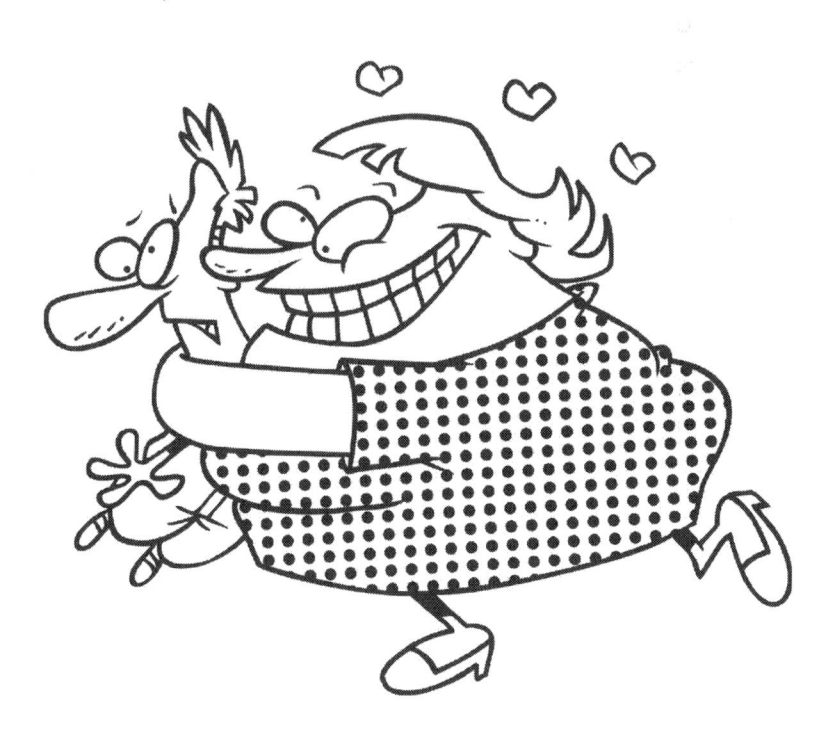

After much thought and mutterings of 'crafty bastards', she came to realise that we were right, and that our knowledge of popular music was much lacking. The message hit home, and armed with this new knowledge, she started to move forward, possibly with the intent of chocking me to death, but instead wrapped her arms around me and started to cry.

ALEX

The patient and the partner

Andrea and his wife Clara came together just 6 months after Andrea's diagnosis.

'I don't know what to do, it's all so frightening, it is so depressing. Tell me what I can do!'

With some surprise I realised it was Clara, and not Andrea, who was talking with tears in her eyes. I told them that it was normal to be anxious, even depressed.

Andrea stirred to life. 'Not for me, I realise I have Parkinson's and that's the way it is.'

Hang on a minute, I thought, it was as if there was a role reversal here. And just to prove it, Clara continued, 'I can't bring myself to tell anybody!'

'I've told all my mates,' chipped in Andrea.

'I can't sleep at night!' was Clara's response.

'I can,' countered Andrea. It was like a ping-pong match, with comments bouncing backwards and forwards, till I finally called time-out.

'Am I correct that it was Andrea who was diagnosed?' I interjected.

'Oh yes! Oh goodness,' and I half expected her to add, 'Oh woe is me,' such was the melodrama.

I couldn't stop a smile, and looking over at Andrea I saw him wink before saying, 'I can handle the Parkinson's but my wife is a different matter.'

I ruefully made a note to contact our psychologist to warn her NOT to give the 'Living with Parkinson's' exercise, as one of the questions in it is 'What five things will you change in your life when you go home.' I felt sure Andrea would put his wife at the top of the list!

The centre's program is designed to help people understand and take control of their lives and their Parkinson's, and to provide fast, effective therapy. Now we were forced to act as referee between the 'patient' and his partner.

At the end of the week, I asked Andrea how he felt. Stupid questions get stupid answers.

'Are you referring to my Parkinson's or my wife?' he answered smiling.

'Well, about both actually!' He was certainly walking better and appeared quite at ease. I couldn't help it, I just had to ask, 'And how does Clara feel?'

His reply was intriguing.

'She reckons if I can improve physically in just 6 days, I can continue to improve, so no big deal.'

We both knew that physical improvement needed daily application, and whilst relieving the symptoms and possibly slowing progression, it was no magic cure.

It was the final day when Clara came over and said, 'I'm sleeping much better and am more at ease about Andrea's situation. Thank you, I am sure I'll be back,'

I assumed she meant with her husband, but couldn't be certain, so I just kissed her on both cheeks and watched them walk out of the centre, the patient and the partner, although which was which I never really knew.

The singing and the songster

Paolo was a slim and tall man who was looking good for his age of 80 years old. He arrived on a fine Sunday in June, and instead of talking to him, I found myself surrounded by his family, all eager to give one particular piece of advice: 'Whatever you do, don't let him sing'.

On this note of wisdom, and with unprecedented speed, they left. There he was alone, looking forlorn and resigned.

'My family are all worried about me,' I thought that indeed they were worried, but not for the reasons he may think.

The warning seemed to prove unnecessary, at least for the first two days, as we saw Paolo gradually gain confidence. It was only when I met him for a one-to-one that I understood that part of his family wished to put him in a home and were encouraging him to 'liquidate his assets'. His daughter in particular was working hard to get a power of attorney over his affairs.

'I don't want to be controlled, but I should listen to them as they have my best interests at heart.' I was sceptical as to whose interest they had at heart but said nothing.

Then the fateful day came, when a call from a local shopkeeper revealed Paolo's secret in all its glory. 'There's a man in the street, I think he is one of yours.' I had not realised we had inherited one. 'He's singing!'

I replied with a simple, 'What?' to which I was informed that he was singing 'O Sole Mio.'

'No, not what song,' I replied. 'What do you mean *in the street*?'

A short pause, followed by the screeching of tires as the reply came through, 'He's literally in the middle of the street.'

I hastened to the scene of the 'crime', to find our local police sitting with him on a park bench. Whilst they were not singing, they were smiling. They told me, 'We have tried to explain to the gentleman that he cannot sing in the middle of the street!'

Paolo tried another approach, 'What if I change the song?'

'No,' came the reply along with a gentle warning.

On their departure, I asked the obvious question. 'What were you doing?'

'Singing!' came the reply. 'Patience', I thought, and then said 'I know that, but why?'

'There were no cars, and it is a lovely day. Everybody seemed to appreciate it!' I had no answer to that.

We of course suspected a psychological problem, and called in our psychologist. Test after test showed remarkable fortitude for a man of 80.

'Sorry,' said our psychologist, followed by some mumbo-jumbo technical words, which I translated as being, 'Repressed with a feeling of being cornered. His singing is just his way of letting it all out.'

We decided to encourage him to sing along quietly to his therapy, as long as he stopped singing in public places. Like a light bulb being turned on, he blossomed both physically and mentally.

On the last day, he lamented, 'What am I going to do when I get home? They'll stop me from singing and I want more liberty. After all, I'm not handicapped; I've just got this Parkinson's thing, and I'm already feeling better!'

'You could always sing in the shower?' I suggested.

'Nope, my daughter lives downstairs and she will hear me!' Strike one.

'In the cellar?'

'Nope, haven't got one.' Strike two. With one last try I offered, 'In a friend's house?'

'Nope, they don't like me going out on my own.'

I felt sorry for him, but he smiled craftily and said, 'I can always sing in the street!'

Oops, I did it again

Carol came to us one Sunday afternoon, with a smile and a small child's scooter, which she used to whizz around on using her stronger leg for propulsion. Her credentials were impeccable as an ex-member of some government, and her husband was well placed in the financial world.

We had no idea what to make of a rich and famous lady flying around on a scooter, but we did know what to make of her Parkinson's. More than 20 years after her diagnosis, she was a packet of raw energy, which we soon focused by giving her ever-harder therapy sessions.

Her blocking (freezing of the muscles) was a major factor, and on one occasion she turned up 30 minutes late with a cheery hello and an 'I got blocked in the lobby' as her explanation. The hotel had 4 stars and was quite upper class; who knows what the other guests thought of seeing her in the lobby, blocked and half standing on a scooter?

She made good progress and made such an impression on me that I agreed to join her with my daughter for dinner. It was raining, and on approaching the lobby, there she was, just 3 metres away, but on the

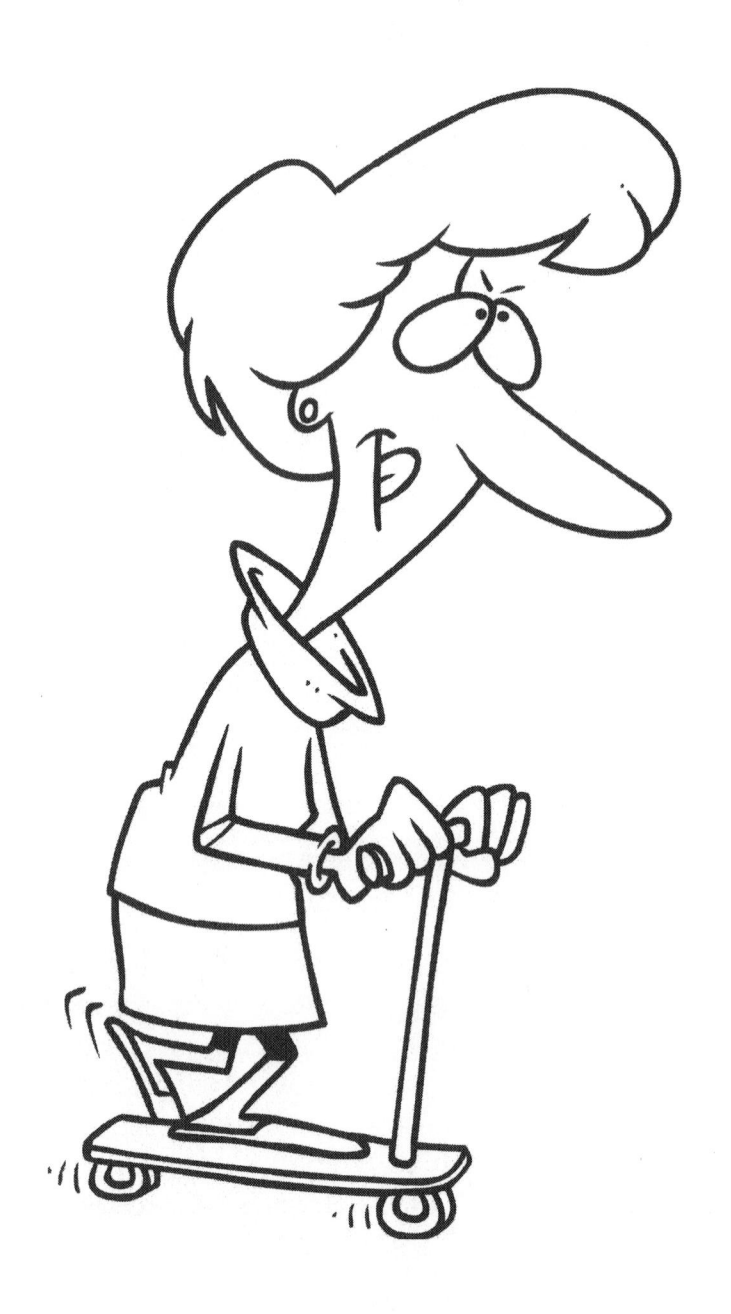

wrong side of the door – and yes, she was blocked. With rain dripping down her face and the scooter abandoned, I prepared my daughter by explaining her that blocking sometimes caused some distress. Nothing could have been further from the truth in this case.

Carol was smiling – not one of those sheepish grins, but a full blossomed, sunshine smile.

'Ooops', she said. 'I'd just popped out and then here we are. I did it again.' She then took pity on my daughter's bemused face and added, 'Blocked, dear. You see, I thought I had more time'.

'Aren't you cold?' enquired my daughter politely.

'Oh no my dear, quite the opposite. I'd been looking forward to a refreshing shower and my clothes needed a wash,' and we all started laughing. 'Help me inside and in 10 minutes I'll be as right as rain.' Well rain did appear to be the appropriate word. We cued her (helped her unblock) and led her to the safety of the lobby.

'My husband gets so annoyed with my blocking,' added Carol.

My daughter replied, 'That's not very nice of him.'

'Oh he is a wonderful man, very sympathetic, he just wished that I didn't block from the neck down. He would much prefer me to block from the neck up and stop talking incessantly,' she replied, winking.

Carol soon became an inspiration and a celebrity in the town. She was unmistakable on her little scooter, charging down the high street and getting waves from people who appeared in shop doors just to greet her with a, 'Buongiorno signora!' and followed by the shouts of pedestrians making rapid moves to avoid collision with a high-speed daredevil who appeared to know no fear.

Our goodbyes were heartfelt, and our time together all too brief. It was as if the town had lost its purpose in the days after she left us. No more smiles, shopkeepers stayed inside, and pedestrians could once again walk the streets without fear.

To be or not to be

Sheila and George were an odd couple. Whilst George was short and robust, Sheila was tall and lanky. Both were in their mid-60s. It was soon apparent that he came to the Centre not on his own volition; as Sheila explained, 'We are here about George's problem.'

His problem, actually, we thought was not so much his Parkinson's, as Sheila herself.

'Poor old George is not coping well, and I have to do everything for him.' This appeared to include all the talking, and we didn't actually get to speak to George until his meeting with the speech therapist. Well, Sheila could hardly do that for him, so poor old George got his moment of liberty to actually talk.

Now, speech therapy for Parkinson's requires using a strong voice reading some classic phrases, even shouting, and I was in a room some 50 metres away when I heard him reciting quite clearly, 'To be or not to be, that is the question.' I thought about it for a minute, and decided it was indeed the question.

For George to be, it meant distracting Sheila. Using our contacts, Sheila suddenly found herself offered a free spa session, a trip to the lake, free massage and other such goodies. In the following days, with Sheila distracted and absent, George told us his remarkable story as an ex-army man and successful businessman and a generally fascinating person. Even more remarkable was his clarity and ability to cope on his own, both physically and mentally. He made little reference to his wife, except to say, 'It makes her happy to be in control.'

Our psychologist asked what made him happy, and it took some time for him to say, 'Fishing,' before adding, 'But I can't do that with Parkinson's.'

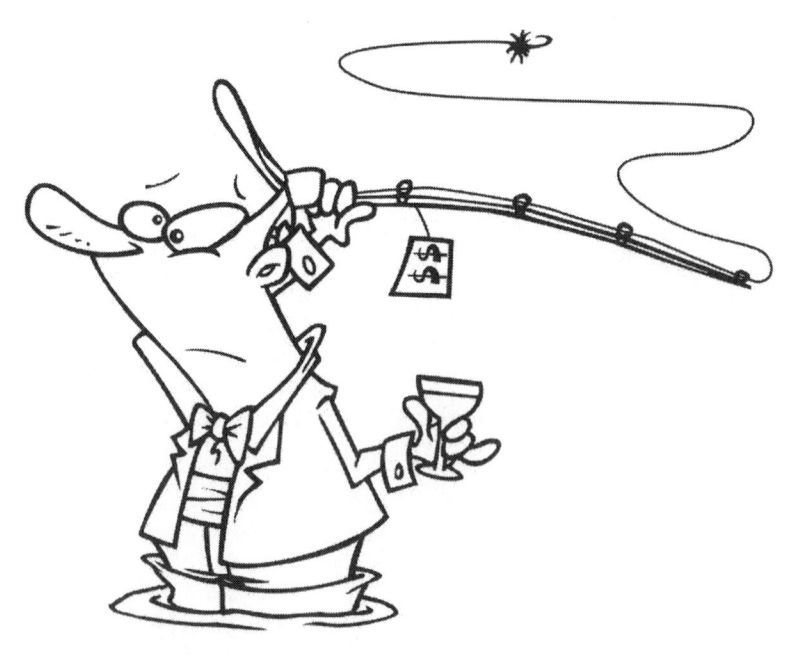

Hmm… sitting on a river bank watching a float bob up and down was well within his abilities, and actually hooking the bait and removing the fish was easily solved as his son enjoyed fishing, too. His son was absolutely delighted to go once a week to the river with his father, but had strong doubts that his mother would 'allow' it.

Sheila was basically a very kind-hearted woman, and it was possibly her excessive devotion to her husband that was the problem. But a plan came together with George now revelling in this new possibility of going fishing with his son.

Sheila came in on the Friday, glowing from her massages, pedicures and spa treatments, and with a wide smile announced that she had been invited to help out at their local Parkinson's centre once a week. 'I've learnt so much from caring for my husband, it's time I gave my knowledge to others.' She said she thought George would be alright for a few hours whilst she popped down to the centre and added, 'The lady even quoted a proverb saying that giving was like fishing, all you need is patience'.

The local Parkinson's centre had a sense of humour. I must remember that if I ever have to suggest something similar. I just hope the next time it's not goose hunting as our goose would be well and truly cooked.

Just call me Bruce

It was some twenty minutes into our first meeting that Simon started to cry.

He was normally a self-contained and quiet man, a landlord of a pub by profession, chairperson of some local political party, member of the local golf club and a pillar of society. His wife looked quite shocked, obviously not used to her pillar falling down.

I waited then asked, 'What's on your mind Simon?' Sometimes this gets a grunt; other times an answer.

No grunt was forthcoming, but after a pause of some 60 seconds, he replied, 'In two years of Parkinson's, nobody had ever told me that I had a full life ahead of me.' This was possibly because he had never asked, never questioned what Parkinson's meant and had assumed the worst.

A dry sense of humour became more and more apparent, as the week went on. Our team found themselves at times baffled (many of them are Italians, and British sarcasm is not understood), at other times amused by the names he adopted for some of the team working closest to him.

It appeared that his personal therapist was now called 'Bruce', referring to Bruce Willis in the *Die Hard* movies, as he never gives up. The irony was that 'Bruce' is a slim, five feet tall girl with long hair, but she played along and even came in one day with a printed T-shirt reading 'Just call me Bruce'.

Simon was absorbing all he could from the various therapists. The pillar was back.

His posture and mood improved greatly, and at the end of the week I asked, 'So what are you going to do differently next week that you didn't do the week before coming here?' I had no idea that he was planning a revolution.

'We will sell the pub and the house, and we are moving to New Zealand for six months.'

His wife was smiling and chipped in, 'We've always wanted to go to New Zealand.'

So three months later, I had an email saying that the final night party at the pub had been a great success, and so many people had turned up that they had needed to hire a marquee. A fortnight after the first message, another email announced their arrival in Auckland. So, pub sold, tick. Dream holiday, tick. End of story, wrong.

Just before Christmas, I got an email with the subject 'Greetings from San Francisco'. My geography is poor, but I know that San Francisco is not in New Zealand, and the email revealed that Paul had 'always wanted to visit America'. And then, after another month, there was a postcard with a maple leaf, which clearly said Canada across the front.

The last mail I had was from Cornwall. It appeared they had taken a pause from seeing the world and opened a bed and breakfast. Why? Well, I didn't need to read the email to know it was something they had 'always wanted to do.'

ALEX

Philosophically speaking

I hardly knew anything about philosophy until we took on a Parkinson's-specialised speech therapist who had first done a degree in philosophy. He would explain a patient's situation with such detail, depth and insight that a patient once replied, 'And I thought I only had Parkinson's!'

Mohammed, a large man with Parkinson's and a master philosopher himself, came to stay with us for two weeks, and as you can imagine, him and our speech therapist immediately found common ground and could often be found having a chat together, although few of us actually understood what they were talking about.

It was towards the end of his stay that I found them in one of our consultation rooms discussing politics, of all things. Mohammed came from a Middle Eastern country that had not seen a change in government in decades. Our speech therapist is from a country that, until recently, had changed it's government on an average of once a year. I decided to steer the conversation onto Parkinson's to see what would happen. Mohammed immediately claimed that he was lucky to have Parkinson's, as it could have been much worse. I knew this line, but asked anyhow what he meant by it.

'I could have been married!' He replied simply. Not the answer I was expecting. 'In my country you don't get to pick your wife, so you never know what to expect, but with Parkinson's, and especially after doing your program, life is much more predictable.'

I decided to ask one of our standard questions.

'What will you do differently when you get back home?'

'I was thinking of taking up astronomy. Much easier to understand than women,' was his reply.

'Do you believe in reading the stars to see our future?' The speech therapist asked.

'No, certainly not,' he exclaimed. 'The light from the stars was actually created thousands of years ago. How can a distant past predict our immediate future?'

I felt we were wandering off topic, so I tried to steer it back again onto Parkinson's, but Mohammed replied, 'I was actually talking about Parkinson's. You see, many of us with Parkinson's look to the past with sadness, and yet want to know the future.' A deep and profoundly true observation.

Mohammed left us on the Sunday with a wave and a parting thought: 'If you could go back in time and know how to avoid Parkinson's, would you do it?'

I smiled. 'No Mohammed, I can't go back in time so the question is just philosophical. I'll stick with having Parkinson's and face reality.'

'You'll never make a great philosopher,' Mohammed grinned. 'But then again you are married.'

ALEX

Grandpa's granddaughter

Paolo initially contacted us by phone and booked for a two-week stay. This in itself was not unusual. The words 'If anybody asks, I'm not booked with you, I'm just on holiday' were perhaps less common.

He arrived on his own; a quiet man, tall with gaunt features and a sad face. He suffered from severe problems with his walking and used a stick, and he didn't really participate in the activities for the first two days, until we finally got him to say what we knew was at the heart of his problem. 'I know I have Parkinson's but I refuse to accept or share it with my family.'

Ah! The 'A' word. Accepting. The battle lines were set.

At the end of the two weeks, his daughter's family came to pick him up, and he told them to meet him on the first floor of the main complex – or in other words, at the therapy centre. They duly arrived and were greeted by Paolo, now walking without a stick, but still with a slight tremor in his left hand.

'I thought it was time to tell you: I've got Parkinson's,' were his first words, even before the hello.

The daughter looked straight at her father and said, 'Dad, we've known that for the last two years. More importantly, how are you?'

He had been practising this moment for days. We had overheard the trial runs of his declaration wafting out of the changing room. He had a speech prepared, and now he was flapping around for words. 'Well that's clear then,' was all he managed.

That evening, Paolo decided a celebratory dinner was needed, so there we all were: Paolo to my left, his daughter in front of him and his granddaughter Clara on the far end to my right. Paolo was nervous, and I knew this not by any great insight but because he stated to me before the dinner, 'I'm nervous about what my daughter is thinking'. But the problem wasn't his daughter's thought process, as I was to find out.

His tremor increased, and he did what all good Parkies do. He sat on the hand. I saw Clara give a little nod of the head, then got up and made her way around the table to her grandfather. She pulled his hand out and said simply, 'Granddad, why do you hide your hand? It doesn't bother me!' and kissed him.

The floodgates opened, as Paolo realised that all his days of hiding and the resultant stress were gone, and all thanks to Clara, who accepted and loved him for who he was. He was better physically, but also better mentally because of a child's love. Yes, our family and those around us suffer in seeing us not feeling too great, but if we let them, they are also part of the solution to that puzzle we call 'Parkinson's.'

Chapter Seven
Humphrey

Humphrey Carpenter

Humphrey is a broadcaster, writer and musician. He was fifty-five when he discovered he had Parkinson's. During his life, he wrote biographies of, among others, JRR Tolkien, WH Auden, Benjamin Britten and Spike Milligan. He wrote children's books: his *Mr Majeika* was televised, and his musical version was performed by the drama group for young people he created in his home city of Oxford – The Mushy Pea Theatre Company. He founded the band Vile Bodies to play 1920s and 30s jazz, and for some time it was the resident band at the *Ritz Hotel* in London. He played bass instruments: tuba, sousaphone, bass saxophone and double bass; it was the double bass that best survived the Parkinson's. He said that the one thing that could make him forget he had Parkinson's was having to play the solid bass beat that a band depends on.

After seeing a comedian performing a one-man show about his progressive MS, Humphrey sketched out his own 'one-man-musical' about Parkinson's, based on well-known songs and entitled 'Shake it all About'. He died (of a heart attack) in 2005 before he could perform it, but he wanted to make Parkinson's funny…

… 'Because believe me, a lot of it is very, very funny.'

Tales of Parkinson's

If you want somebody to give up their seat (say on the tube or the train) you need to carry a walking stick, otherwise people may not realise you are disabled. They may, however, think you are drunk. This happened to me twice. Once in a Turkish restaurant, and then when I turned up to play in a band at our local community centre, and was told that Alcoholics Anonymous were the next door down.

But should you carry one or two walking sticks? Those telescopic mountain poles that have become so fashionable with middle-aged fell-walkers are ideal for Parkinson's. But I for one don't care to look like a mountaineer when heading along Upper Regent Street towards the BBC.

Then there's the threat of the wheelchair. Or is it a golden future, being like a Paralympic athlete whizzing around the place? On the odd occasions I've been in a wheelchair at airports I've tended to be used as a battering ram. Or there was the time I visited the Edward Hopper exhibition at the Tate Modern, and I borrowed one of their electric buggies to go round in comfort. Unfortunately, I had just taken a Pramipexole, and it made me drop off to sleep every few seconds. The consequence was that I kept bumping into people. I think I ran over somebody's foot – and worse still, I woke at one moment to find myself heading at high speed for one of the biggest pictures. It might even have been *Night Hawks* itself, which reaches nearly to the floor.

Halfway up the stairs is a place where I freeze.

Freezing is something that the rest of the world, who don't have Parkinson's, simply don't know about, even if they have been told. You can't know about it unless you have experienced it – it's so silly it seems unbelievable. Freezing is when you come to a complete halt, and can't get going again for quite a long while, maybe half a minute, maybe a lot more. To some extent, it's controllable by Levodopa, as the freezing is caused by low levels of dopamine, and the pill restores that. Last time I had a freeze, my mobile rang in the next room, where I had left it, and I got there all right before it was diverted to the message service. But when I wanted to come back into the study, nothing happened. I was simply pinned to the spot, unable to move, or at least lacking what suddenly seemed like a huge area of skill and experience – the complicated mechanism which allows one to carry out one's own decisions. *Sorry, out of order.* And then it all comes back again, movement returns, decision-making connects itself up to the muscles once again, and – hey presto! – I'm on my way back to the computer, not having lost very much time.

It took me two and half hours to get up and get dressed one morning:

Slow down, you move too fast,
Got to make the morning last...

Puttin' on my socks

This is a song that has to be sung to the tune of Puttin' on the Ritz.

I woke up at crack of dawn,
What a lovely sunny morn.
I'll put on my Sunday best,
See how quickly I'll get dressed!

T-shirt just takes a minute,
There's really nothing in it.
I'll be looking so neat --
But wait! I've forgotten my feet.

The hardest thing I have to do
Each morning when I'm racing
Against the clocks –
Putting on my socks!

First of all, the left one --
This used to be the deft one,
But now it's full of rocks -
Putting on my socks!

HUMPHREY

Socks should be much easier than buttons,
Or a welly,
But they are invisible to gluttons,
Behind the belly.

Hours and hours go past in a trice,
My feet have both turned to ice,
Or wooden blocks,
Puttin' on my socks!

In a perfect world we'd go barefoot,
There, foot, why won't you move?
It jams, it locks,
Puttin' on my socks.

Now I've really done them, but look,
The buggers! they're full of holes,
And the clock tick-tocks,
Puttin' on my socks!

Chapter Eight
Andrew & Esther

Andrew Leach

Andrew was born in London and has been married to Esther for 40 years. They are the proud parents of 2 children, which, in his words, are his greatest achievement as they turned out to be "a bit of alright". He was diagnosed with Parkinson's 4 years ago and lives in hope of a cure within his lifetime, but is not holding his breath.

Esther Leach

Esther is the wife of a Parkie, but certainly does not see herself as a "carer". She was born in Switzerland and her children are bilingual, speaking both English and German, much to the frustration of her husband who has never mastered German. She dreamt of becoming an archeologist but actually was a conference organiser. She loves knitting and travelling.

ANDREW AND ESTHER

Andrew
My Life as a Guinea Pig

I joined my last employer when I was 27 years old, so by the time I reached 60 I had worked there for over 30 years. It had been a big part of my life, maybe too big. I loved much of my work. I loved the camaraderie with my colleagues – some of us had worked together for decades. I loved some of the technical challenges, as during those years I had developed a reputation for solving technical problems, which had spread in the company way beyond the UK. Sure, there was sometimes a lot of stress and I found that increasingly difficult to cope with, but the things I loved greatly outweighed those that I didn't like so much.

Then the company decided to close the plant I had worked at for all those years, so I had no choice; my life at work was coming to an end. I was due to retire on 1st April, a suitable date to start a new life.

Two months before that date, I was diagnosed with Parkinson's. I wasn't expecting that – who does? But, being a scientist, I decided I'd better find out a bit about this condition, since it seemed I was stuck with it for the rest of my life. Like anyone with a new condition, the first thing you do is search on the Internet, where you find a myriad of sites providing vast amounts of information and you have to try and sift through it. I looked on the Parkinson's UK website and made contact with my local group. At the first meeting there was a talk by a local researcher, which got me thinking, 'That could be interesting...' So I looked for local research studies who were looking for volunteers. That took me to Oxford and the Oxford Parkinson's Disease Centre, where I signed up for the Discovery project.

As I found further projects wanting volunteers, I found I couldn't resist – was it the drugs? Can you become a compulsive guinea pig? Soon you realise that there are only a limited number of tests and you can do: finger tapping, toe tapping, being told to relax while my arms are moved around to test for rigidity (always tough that one, I don't do 'relax' very well, especially when someone is trying to take control of one of my limbs).

I was asked if I would donate some skin cells and some cerebral fluid for research. My wife was horrified at the thought of me having a lumbar puncture, convinced I could end up in a wheelchair – I think medical science has moved on a bit on that. Giving skin cells was a fascinating thought: these can be turned into stem cells and hence into neurons, or any other cells researchers need to study. Which means long after I've

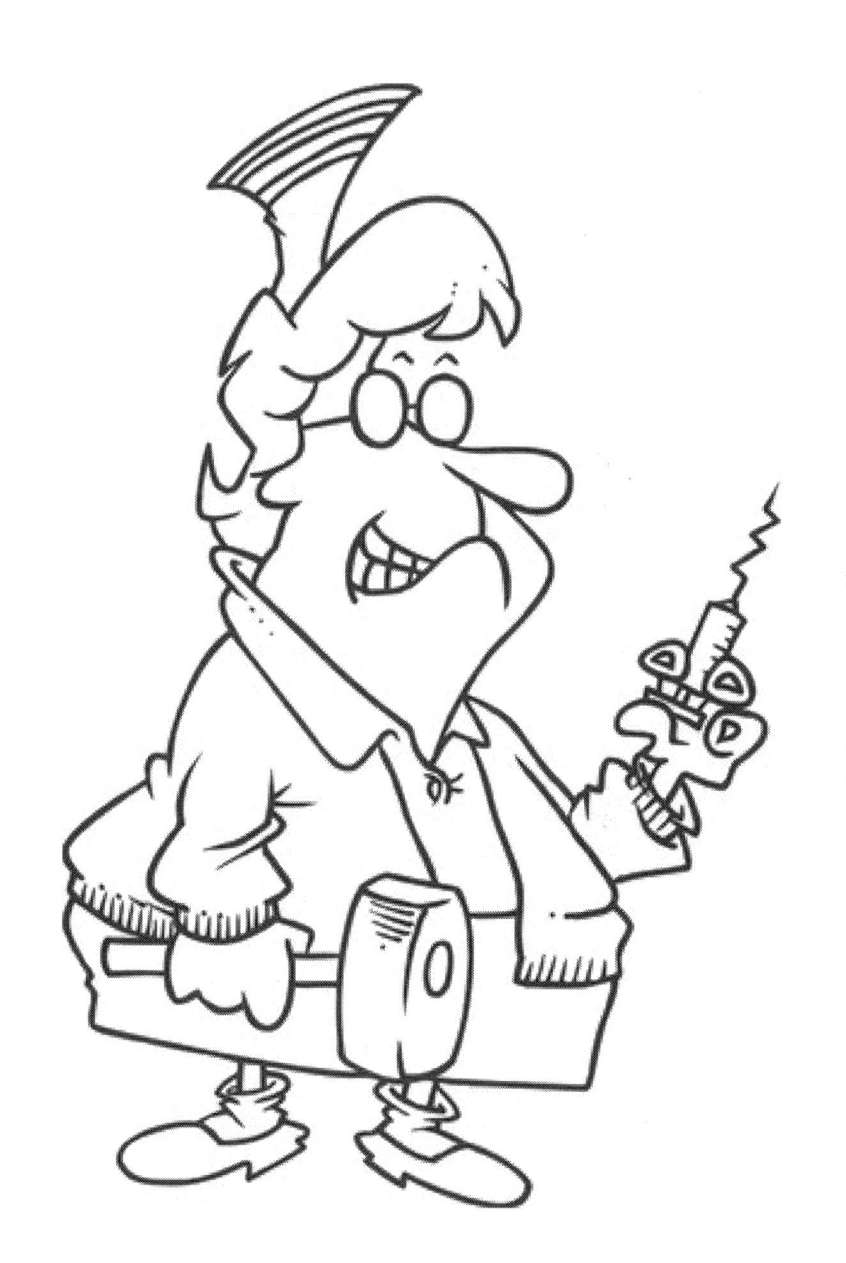

shuffled off this mortal coil there could be bits of me sitting in laboratories around the world!

So one sunny afternoon we sat in the foyer of the John Radcliffe Hospital in Oxford, waiting to be greeted by the researcher who was going to take these samples. I pointed to someone on the other side of the lobby.

'That's got to be him,' I said to my wife.

'It can't be,' she replied. 'He looks like he's only just left school!'

Well it was and he hadn't, and he took the skin biopsy and carried out the lumbar puncture without a hitch (and without any pain!). I wonder what bits of me they have managed to grow in their Petri dishes – whatever they are, I hope they are useful.

Since most of the tests used in the trials are the same as I did in the previous ones, you'd think that would skew the results after a while, but fortunately my short term memory is pretty weak now, so I can't really remember what I said last time. Although I wish I could find the pot of gold at the end of the rainbow that seems to be included in the standard text for every neurological speech test I've undertaken.

Then again, why is it that, when asked to choose a rating out of 1, 2, 3, 4 and 5, I always want to select 2.75 or 3.25? Does Parkinson's make you even more perverse than before, or does it just make it harder to make a decision?

So, for the first two years after diagnosis, I volunteered for a total of 17 research studies, but these were all what the Americans call observational studies – none of these were clinical trials, where a new drug or therapy is tested (often called Interventional studies in the USA). I now felt it was time to find a clinical trial and discovered that there was a trial starting at the National Hospital for Neurology in London involving an existing diabetes drug called Exenatide. I went for the assessment, was accepted and became number 9 – which was disappointing, as I had really wanted to be number 6. Then I realised that this meant that, for 48 weeks of my life, I would have to inject myself with what may be a drug or may just be a (very expensive) saline solution. Now, at this point I should point out that I do suffer from one other medical condition – abject cowardice! But I was trapped, so every Wednesday I had to steel myself to mix up the potion and push the needle into the fat round my tummy – fortunately there's a fair amount of that to aim for.

So, why did I do it? It's interesting! You meet lots of very skilled and usually very pleasant researchers, who know a lot about your condition and often have more time to talk about issues than your regular medical advisers. Yes, you have to give samples of blood, undergo all sorts of tests, maybe have more scans, give more blood, have a lumbar puncture, give even more blood (we were once just leaving the National Hospital after a full morning of tests when the senior research nurse came running out shouting 'Andrew, come back, I need more blood!' – but he was so charming, I could forgive him anything!), but every time you learn more and more about this condition you have. Of course, in the back of your mind you always hope that you will help bring forward that 'magic bullet', which will bring an end to Parkinson's, but you know the chances of that are pretty small.

Everyone thinks of people with Parkinson's having a shuffling walk and shaking a lot. But there are so many other issues we have to contend with. One early issue for me was politely described once as "urinary urgency". That doesn't sound too bad – you just need to pee suddenly, but combine that with a loss of fine motor control, which make it much more difficult to undo buttons and zips quickly – nature has a cruel streak sometimes!

Talking of incontinence, there are lots of good products out there which can help – pads and pants and so on. It's not a subject for polite conversation, but if they help make life easier, that's fine by me. But tell me, why do supermarkets insist on hiding men's products in the middle of the section labelled something like 'feminine intimate hygiene'? Next time you see a man peering furtively amongst a myriad of tampons, don't assume he's got some strange perversion, he's probably just got Parkinson's.

Mae West is quoted as asking, 'Is that a gun in your pocket, or are you just pleased to see me?' Sadly these days, it's more likely to be my incontinence pad.

When I was young, I wanted to make the earth move, these days, I happy if I can just get a decent bowel movement... ah well!

Esther
Midnight Snacks

My husband has always had a sweet tooth, and although I used to hide the chocolates and other goodies in high cupboards so that the children could not help themselves, my husband certainly could reach them and had a knack of tracking down their hiding places. I would berate him every time, but his addiction was too far gone.

The kids have long grown up and left the nest now, but my husband's search for the treasured sweets has continued. Since getting Parkinson's he has become more crafty, and knowing I would give him a hard time if I caught him, he has taken to creeping around the house after midnight.

At first I got quite a fright hearing strange noises coming up the stairs in the early hours of the morning, but I soon worked out that the noises were from my husband's undercover hobby of hunting down the midnight snack of hidden sweets. Even the garage door got opened, and on more than one occasion, I distinctly heard the moving of furniture and rustling of curtains.

The morning after he would act normally and admit nothing even when confronted with chocolate-stained curtains and a trail of crumbs leading out of the sitting room and ending directly beside his part of the bed.

His innocent face suggested that the evidence had been planted and he was being framed, but then he would give me a gorgeous smile. No confession was ever given and I never sought one – after all, who could resist that smile and who could not love him for his dedication to the task. I now hide chocolate bars, popcorn and even hot cross buns in the darkest recesses of the house each night just before going to bed, just so my husband could find them and give me that gorgeous smile every morning.

Conclusion by Alexander Reed, director of the European Parkinson Therapy Centre

We all have a degenerative condition in us called ageing, yet most people of 70 years do not blame their age for their reduced ability to do things. When we have Parkinson's, this accepting and adapting to this reality is harder, as we are less prepared for it. But nevertheless, we must adapt, and as with old age, accept that we are simply less able.

Our health services in Europe are also not always in our favour. We get the diagnosis, a packet of pills and an appointment somewhere down the line. It comes as a shock to the system and it is little understood that it is a shock to the family, too. What are we meant to do? What is going to happen? We feel like a beached whale with the tide going out.

It is fundamental to understand that Parkinson's affects the whole family, and the whole family needs support and reassurance.

It's not surprising that over 50% of people with Parkinson's are clinically depressed, and that the vast majority do not seek help, but head for the nearest desk and hide under it, figuratively speaking! The sad truth about Parkinson's is that the real truth is never made clear.

I wish that when first diagnosed I had been told; 'You can reduce symptoms by up to 40%; you can help slow progression, and your life will become more precious, not less, if you make the right choices'.

Some of us are reluctant to admit that we have Parkinson's, almost as if we are afraid to be looked upon as different or weaker. Yet even the person who comes last in an event in the Paralympics is applauded, because he or she has chosen to fight. Anybody who faces adversity with determination is stronger for it.

Words like 'Parkinson's made me a better man' or 'Parkinson's was an opportunity' make little sense at that moment of diagnosis.

According to one famous study (*Parkinson's Outcomes Project*), the number one thing that destroys the quality of life of a person with Parkinson's is apathy and depression, and not all the usual suspects that are related to motor functions. This point is essential in learning to live with Parkinson's.

Time and time again, I meet families devastated by Parkinson's, and week in and week out we explain that Parkinson's may bring a change of life, but sometimes that change can actually strengthen the family and be a new opportunity for your life. Parkinson's does not destroy our lives, it just means we must adapt to the limits it imposes.

Our therapy model is based on the concept that there are four key elements (what we call 'pillars') to maintain quality of life. Medicines are of course at the core, but like a house with one wall, it will not keep the roof up. Medicines to a depressed person will not change his or her life. You need all four pillars delivered in one place intensively.

If you want to learn a foreign language, one hour per week will not work. Two weeks of full-immersion will have a much higher impact - and even more so if you apply what you have learned and speak that language every day for the rest of your life. It is the same for Parkinson's, an appointment here and a dance class there will not be enough to change our quality of life.

So, what are the four pillars of Parkinson's?

Medicine

Medicine, as we previously mentioned, is what keeps us moving and eases some aspects of Parkinson's. One well-known British neurologist told me recently, 'We know a lot about Parkinson's, but we don't and can't know what is truly like to *have* Parkinson's'. This is a remarkable insight, and probably why this neurologist is so exceptional.

I have seen many people who have visited over 10 different Neurologists and complain that they have not found the right one who can 'solve' their problems. It is unrealistic that in a 20-minute appointment a Neurologist can solve all the complex issues surrounding Parkinson's with a pill. Medicine is an essential pillar not a crutch.

Physical movement

Physical movement is now understood better. Like taking pills, it is now scientifically accepted that it must be done daily to see and maintain results. Regularity is better than quantity. But what must we do to improve our condition with movement? Walking is a basic and fundamental aspect of daily life with Parkinson's. It produces a neuro-protective effect; in short, it helps slow down neuro-degeneration, which is good for everybody, but especially for those of us with Parkinson's.

Tango therapy, going to the gym and physiotherapy are often mentioned, but in reality, if not done regularly, they have limited effect, but can be fun, which certainly is a plus.

Studies show that physiotherapy needs to be combined with conscious thought: 'Think before you move.' This point is often missed and is based on the concept of neuroplasticity. If someone breaks a leg, they may do physiotherapy, but for us the problem is inside our head, so physiotherapy must be combined with conscious thought. If we think and correct our posture, length of stride and arm movement, and then actually consciously keep doing it, we find that over a short period of time the brain adapts and this correction becomes automatic. Rather like if you always sleep on your side, and one day, because you have a broken rib, you are forced to sleep on our back. For the first few nights this probably means little sleep, but then our brain accepts the new reality, and even after the rib is healed, you continue to sleep happily on your back.

Group therapy is popular too, but everybody is different in his or her Parkinson's. Take four chefs and give them the same ten ingredients, and you'll end up with four different meals. If you really want to reduce your symptoms, you need to work individually with a specialist to identify, correct and learn to maintain this correction.

Lifestyle

Lifestyle is perhaps the least understood, and hence the less treated of the four pillars. Apart from well-known points about what and when we eat and the avoidance and management of stress, what is essential to understand is that we have a choice in how we live our lives. We can choose to be apathetic and negative, or we can choose to take control. We can choose to delegate our quality of life to medicines or to our spouses, or we can choose to focus our lives on doing what we can enjoy. Choosing to continue at full speed is not a choice; it is denial. Full speed is like driving a car fast with an engine that is slowly losing power; at some stage it will break down. Life will change, but who says we cannot decide how it should change? If we choose to do less but do more of what we enjoy, then our quality of life is maintained. We often confuse quantity with quality of life.

Psychology

We use the ACMA approach. The first step is to ACCEPT we have Parkinson's; that means accepting something we don't want, but just like ageing, it is a fact. How can we fight something if we do not accept it exists? Like going into a boxing ring with a blindfold, we are going to get hit hard. Take the blindfold off, and hit back!

COMPREHENSION of the reality of Parkinson's makes us stronger, as we realise we can influence progression and symptoms. It's much harder to fight a war we do not believe in or one in which we do not understand the strategy. Only if we accept and comprehend it can we be MOTIVATED, and this will only be effective if we combine what we need to do with what we enjoy doing. We cannot stay motivated if we are always doing things we have to do with no reward. Dopamine is released into our brain when we do something enjoyable, so we become more inclined to take a long, healthy walk if, for instance, it brings us a reward like a stop at an ice cream shop or your local pub.

These three stages bring about real ACTION, which we can sustain and believe in. Too many people talk about what we must do (the action), without having accepted, understood and decided to actually do it.

If one of the above pillars goes down, it may pull down the others too. That's why apathy and depression are so destructive. If we stop caring, we stop exercising and we stop living. We are then left with just the medicines – back to square one – and worse, we enter what one leading neurologist called 'The Vortex of Apathy'. The vortex pulls us down, eliminates neuroprotection and neuroplasticity, and it destroys people with Parkinson's and the lives of those around them.

Looking back at what we were able to do before Parkinson's instead of all the things we can still do is at the root of many people's depression. Looking forward, we may experience fear and anxiety. 'Where will I be in ten years? What does the future hold?' All of this put together can create the apathy so associated with Parkinson's. The truth is that neither looking backwards or forwards is relevant. It is today that is relevant, and we should focus on managing and maximising our lives every day: seeing the funny side, learning the truth and living a full life with Parkinson's.

People with Parkinson's have a simple request: we need support, not as patients, but as people and families.

This book is written by people with Parkinson's. It is a window into the lives of people who truly know what quality of life means. They also know that seeing the funny side is essential, and through sharing such experiences, the strange puzzle that we call Parkinson's is made real and relevant to all of us.

CONCLUSION

Since this book was written

The European Parkinson Therapy Centre (EuPaTh) has had a notable resonance throughout Italy and also abroad (From Australia, Singapore, Japan, Venezuala, USA and of course Europe) is active all year round and has brought many people to stay in Boario's hotels in this unusually beautiful part of Italy, with 5 lakes, Europe's largest in-land island, riverside towns, mountains and valleys.

Now members of The European Parkinson Disease Association (EPDA), the centres' unique approach is changing lives and changing the way people with Parkinson's are treated. What most distinguishes Eupath are its dedicated and sensitive staff.

"Thank you very much for everything you have done for us and for my dad. You have been fantastic and professional. The sensitivity and humanity you give to your patients is priceless and moving. For Alex I have no adjectives. He too experiences the difficulties of this disease every day, but he is a real warrior and prefers to dedicate most of his time to his clients rather than just thinking about himself. You are a half miracle. " (Franco from Rome)

Given the centre's reputation, it has been possible to add a new building for vocational training, which includes a fully equipped web Studio broadcasting and involving thousands of people per week and a professional training center (online and classroom) to train health professionals on the treatment of Parkinson's disease the EuPaTh way: dignity, self-empowerment, real results, motivation, multilevel, so that the centre's innovative approach can spread across Europe.

People with Parkinson's are remarkable people not patients, with great courage and strength. We dedicate this book especially to them.

With special thanks to:
Dr. Becky Farley and PWR moves
Dr. Barbara Borroni and Dr. Marinella Turla
and the Terme di Boario, Italy

References

European Parkinson's Therapy Centre
Specialised Parkinson's rehabilitation centre

www.parkinsontherapy.com
info@parkinsontherapy.com

Parkinson's UK
The Parkinson's charity that drives better care, treatments and quality of life

www.parkinsons.org.uk
hello@parkinsons.org.uk
0808 800 0303

The Cure Parkinson's Trust
Fund research to slow, stop or reverse Parkinson's

www.cureparkinsons.org.uk
cptinfo@cureparkinsons.org.uk
020 7487 3892